Praise for *Complete Care for Your Aging Dog*

"I'm a veteran veterinarian, but I learned an incredible amount about the caring for an aging pet in Shojai's groundbreaking book. . . . To borrow a phrase from an old dog food commercial, this book is so complete, all you add is love!"

—Dr. Marty Becker, resident veterinarian on
Good Morning America and author of
The Healing Power of Pets

"Need a quick reference? *Complete Care for Your Aging Dog* provides a practical, easy-to-read guide about health care for the aging dog. If you have an aging dog, this is a must-read book. It provides simple question-and-answer treatment of essentials of aging dogs."

—Johnny D. Hoskins, DVM, Ph.D., and
internist for older dogs and cats

Praise for Amy D. Shojai's *Pet Care in the New Century*

"Thoughtful, groundbreaking, and often inspirational . . . an important work that everyone who cares about pets and the future of veterinary medicine must read."

—Gina Spadafori, author of *Dogs for Dummies*

"A worthwhile addition to the library of dog and cat owners."
—*Bellwether*, News Magazine of the University
of Pennsylvania Journal of Veterinary
Medicine

"Wow! After thirty-one years of practice, I am amazed that a person can create a book that covers all aspects of modern veterinary care. This book will prove to be an invaluable resource to companion animal lovers, students, and the profession. I am in awe that Ms. Shojai has been able to pull so many people together in this work."

—Robert A. Taylor, DVM, seen on
TV's *Emergency Vets*

continued . . .

"Amy Shojai delivers cutting-edge medicine with more flair than Emeril Lagasse, presenting the amazing array of astonishing advances in veterinary medicine. If you have a pet with heart disease, cancer, kidney failure—or any other serious medical condition—this easy to comprehend book is a credible place to start for your research. Shojai continues to rank among the most authoritative and thorough pet reporters."

—Steve Dale, syndicated newspaper columnist of
My Pet World and host of the radio programs
Animal Planet Radio and *Pet Central*

Praise for Amy D. Shojai's *Complete Kitten Care*

"What baby expert Dr. Benjamin Spock did for people, kitten expert Amy Shojai has done for cats. . . . Everything you need to know to begin a blissful life with your kitty."

—Ed Sayres, president, San Francisco SPCA

"When you purchase a kitten, there should be four requirements by law: food, water dish, litter box, and this book."

—Steve Dale, *Pet Central* radio host
and syndicated columnist

"Finally there's an informative, fun-filled guide to help us raise the best cats possible . . . filled with practical solutions, delightful stories, and the latest in kitten-care research."

—Bob Walker and Frances Mooney, authors of
The Cats' House and *Cats into Everything*

"Covers kitten selection and care issues from A to Z . . . [a] thorough guide to getting your new baby off on the right paw."

—Carole Nelson Douglas, author of
the Midnight Louie mysteries

"Another great book from Amy Shojai. . . . *Complete Kitten Care* should be as important to the owner as kitten food is to the kitten."

—Bob Vella, host of nationally syndicated
Pet Talk America and author of *300 Incredible
Things for Pet Lovers on the Internet*

"A wealth of information for first-time kitten owners. Amy Shojai shows you how to enjoy kittenhood."

> —Pam Johnson-Bennett, feline behaviorist
> and author of *Think Like a Cat*
> and *Psycho Kitty?*

"*Complete Kitten Care* will give you all the information you need to successfully grow your young feline. Informative and fun to read."

> —John C. Wright, Ph.D., certified applied
> animal behaviorist and author of
> *Is Your Cat Crazy?*

"A must-have for anyone considering kittenhood. . . . This books covers it all, from selecting a compatible kitten to handling emergencies, in a comprehensive and understandable manner."

> —H. Ellen Whiteley, DVM, author of
> *Understanding and Training Your Cat or Kitten*

"Thorough, entertaining and authoritative . . . a primer on the feline mystique, one that owners are sure to turn to again and again as their kitten grows into cathood."

> —Kim Thornton, president, Cat Writers' Association

"Amy Shojai has once again given the cat-loving public a concise, easy-to-understand book. I wish it could accompany every kitten going to a new home."

> —Kitty Angell, secretary, Cat Fanciers' Association Inc.

"Amy Shojai, the doyenne of pet care books, has come up with another winner. There's something here for everyone, whether you're a newbie at kitten care or an old pro. This book is an extremely comprehensive resource that will ensure selection of your perfect kitten and guide you in helping him become a happy, healthy, lifelong companion."

> —Sally Bahner, freelance writer and feline expert

Other NAL books by Amy D. Shojai

COMPLETE CARE FOR YOUR AGING CAT

COMPLETE KITTEN CARE

PET CARE IN THE NEW CENTURY:
Cutting-Edge Medicine for Dogs and Cats

COMPLETE CARE FOR

Your Aging Dog

AMY D. SHOJAI

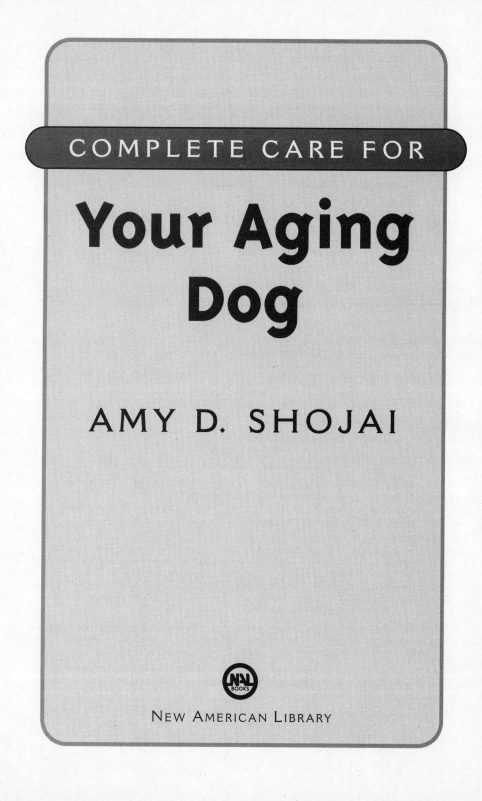

NEW AMERICAN LIBRARY

NEW AMERICAN LIBRARY
Published by New American Library, a division of
Penguin Group (USA) Inc., 375 Hudson Street, New York, New York 10014, U.S.A.
Penguin Books Ltd, 80 Strand, London WC2R 0RL, England
Penguin Books Australia Ltd, 250 Camberwell Road, Camberwell, Victoria 3124, Australia
Penguin Books Canada Ltd, 10 Alcorn Avenue, Toronto, Ontario, Canada M4V 3B2
Penguin Books (N.Z.) Ltd, Cnr Rosedale and Airborne Roads, Albany, Auckland, 1310, New Zealand

Penguin Books Ltd, Registered Offices: 80 Strand, London WC2R 0Rl, England

First published by New American Library, a division of Penguin Group (USA) Inc.

First Printing, July 2003
1 3 5 7 9 10 8 6 4 2

LIBRARY OF CONGRESS CATALOGING-IN-PUBLICATION DATA:
Shojai, Amy, 1956–
Complete care for your aging dog / Amy D. Shojai.
p. cm.
Includes bibliographical references (p.).
ISBN 0-451-20789-0 (alk. paper)
1. Dogs.   2. Dogs—Aging.   3. Dogs—Diseases.   4. Veterinary geriatrics.   I. Title.

SF427 .S556 2003
636.7'089897—dc21
2002041059

Set in New Caledonia
Designed by Eve L. Kirch

Printed in the United States of America

PUBLISHER'S NOTE
Every effort as been made to ensure that the information contained in this book is complete and accurate. However, neither the publisher nor the author is engaged in rendering professional advice or services to the individual reader. The ideas, procedures, and suggestions contained in this book are not intended as a substitute for consulting with your pet's physician. All matters regarding your pet's health require medical supervision. Neither the author nor the publisher shall be liable or responsible for any loss or damage allegedly arising from any information or suggestion in this book.

While the author has made every effort to provide accurate telephone numbers and Internet addresses at the time of publication, neither the publisher nor the author assumes any responsibility for errors, or for changes that occur after publication.

For Fafnir—

Thirteen years were not enough.

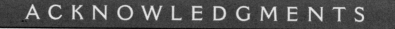
ACKNOWLEDGMENTS

Many individuals helped make this book a reality by sharing their expertise, help, and inspirational pet stories. My husband, Mahmoud, my caring and supportive family, and my dear friends remind me daily of what's truly important. You all know who you are—and I can't thank y'all enough.

My colleagues from the Dog Writers Association of America, Cat Writers' Association, and other "pet fanciers" never fail to inspire and impress me with their professionalism and support. I'd especially like to thank Janine Adams, Deb Eldredge, Carol Freeman, Karen Henry, Stacy Pober, Lyn Richards, Debby Rothman, Lynne Rutenberg, Susan Vite, Michelle West, and Stephen Zink for sharing a few of their expert sources, especially for the E-lists and on-line health care contacts. This book was born at The Writer's BBS International Writers Community (www.writersbbs.com) when answering a question about book proposals gave me the idea. It seems that the Furry Muse strikes with inspiration in many places.

The many "Golden Moments" add so much to the book. Thank you to Janine Adams, Kent Foster, Tina Horton, Pam Gauthier, Carole Kjellsen, Nancy Lind, Gail Mirabella, Ellen Ponall, Anne Rassios, Madelene Rutz, and Gina Spadafori for sharing these lovely stories about your special dogs. I am touched by your generosity.

Heartfelt appreciation goes to the many veterinarians and pet professionals who allowed me to report their groundbreaking therapies for aging dogs. I must also thank the countless veterinary schools and specialty colleges who put me in touch with these experts and pet owners, most particularly the American Veterinary Medical Association; Tania Banak of the University of Wisconsin—Madison; Chris Beuoy of the University of Illinois; Cheryl May of Kansas State University; Cynthia K. Ebbers of the American College of Veterinary Internal Medicine; Pat Edwards of Louisiana State University; Lynn Narlesky of the University of California—Davis; Lisa Sigler and Chuck Montera of the American College of Veterinary Surgeons; and Derek Woodbury of the American Animal Hospital Association. The wide range of experts you suggested helped give this book wonderful credibility—I am in your debt.

Grateful thanks once again to my editor, Ellen Edwards. Sincere appreciation and admiration go to my agent, Meredith Bernstein, who does all the really hard stuff so I can live my pet-writing dream.

Finally, this book wouldn't be possible without all the special dogs that share our hearts—and the loving owners dedicated to providing the best care possible for their aging furry family members. Without you, this book would never have been written.

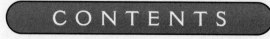

CONTENTS

PART TWO: A-TO-Z HEALTH CONCERNS

PART THREE: ADDITIONAL RESOURCES

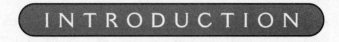
INTRODUCTION

There has been a paradigm shift in the way people treat their dogs. We have become a nation of pet lovers—more than a third of U.S. households keep dogs. No longer are they thought of as mere pets; 70 percent of owners consider their pets to be part of their family. Consequently, there has been a greater focus on wellness care extended to furry family members.

A lifetime of better care means dogs today live longer, healthier lives than ever before. In the past fifty years, the average life span of small dogs has nearly tripled. They used to live to be only six or seven years old, but today many Toy breeds live into their late teens or early twenties. Even large-breed dogs, which age more quickly, have doubled their life span in the past few decades. For example, today it's not unusual for a German Shepherd to reach ten to thirteen years of age, whereas in the past a seven-year-old shepherd was considered ancient.

Today, 40 percent of all pet owners have an animal aged seven or older. What has prompted this shift to an aged pet population? For one thing, dogs used to spend most of their time outside with little or no supervision. Consequently, dogs became victims of extremes of temperature, malice from disgruntled neighbors, exposure to disease, and accidental injuries that cut their lives short.

For example, dogs of the past were typically infested with a variety of disease-causing parasites, which also made them more susceptible to other illnesses and less able to recover. Viral diseases such as distemper and parvovirus killed 50 percent or more of dogs before their first birthday. Repeated pregnancies without proper nutritional support also caused early death to the mother dogs, and produced offspring that often were unable to survive past puppyhood. Roaming and squabbling over breeding issues resulted in debilitating fight injuries among adults, and if a dog's behavior became a problem, he was put to death. Being hit by a car was also a top cause of early canine death. Even when dogs survived, owners often were unable or unwilling to treat the injuries, in part because dogs were considered to be replaceable. People simply put the injured or sick dog to sleep, then got another pet and didn't think much about it.

Until the last decade, few dogs lived long enough to suffer from "old dog" conditions such as arthritis or cataracts. Those that did were rarely treated, either because owners weren't interested, or the veterinary community hadn't yet developed the ability to diagnose and treat such things on a routine basis.

Today, dogs are living longer primarily because owners take better care of them. Most pet dogs live at least part of the time inside the house with their human family, and when outside, they are supervised or kept safe inside fenced yards. Many dogs receive at least some basic training, and owners seek behavior help if problems develop.

Secondly, dogs are living longer because better veterinary treatments are now available, and are routinely sought by owners. Dogs receive preventive medications to guard against deadly pests such as heartworms, intestinal parasites, ticks, and fleas. Highly effective vaccinations for distemper developed in the 1960s, and for parvovirus in the early 1980s, prevent the early deaths of dogs from these diseases. Highly palatable and nutritious dog foods support the animal's physical health to develop healthy bones, muscles, and immune system.

Modern breeders study the science and genetics of reproduction to ensure that they produce healthy pedigreed animals that live longer. Spaying and neutering of pet dogs at an early age has become the norm. This eliminates potential behavior problems as well as health issues, such as breast cancer, and helps to increase the life span of dogs.

Finally, dogs are living longer because many pet owners choose to treat chronic conditions such as arthritis and diabetes, and are able and willing to offer a wide range of treatment and home care to keep aging dogs healthy, happy, and active. Rather than car accidents or viruses that cut lives short, modern dogs more typically succumb to diseases such as cancer, or heart or kidney failure that tend to strike after age ten. Modern treatments help maintain the dog's quality of life, and this better care translates into extra years of enjoyment people can share with their special dogs.

Extra years together mean the loving bond people share with dogs becomes even stronger as time goes by. Older dogs also offer benefits—steadiness, known behaviors and temperament, calm demeanor—which pups may take years to develop. For instance, children may grow up with a special dog that serves as a best friend; then as the dog ages, he evolves into a nonjudgmental trusted confidant during the child's turbulent teenage years. A dog may be the one familiar constant in families split apart by divorce, offering stress relief to both the adults and children involved.

Oftentimes, a young or middle-aged dog accompanies his youthful owner to college, and then travels down the aisle with her (sometimes literally!) when she marries and begins her new family. A graying older dog often "adopts" human babies in the family as her own, and serves as protector, playmate, and even a furry security blanket to the infant. Aging dogs can also give a new purpose and fill the void left in the household when children go away to college, or if the death of a spouse leaves the surviving person bereft.

USING THIS BOOK

Your veterinarian is, of course, an excellent source of information about your aging dog's needs. Many times, though, he or she will have only a limited amount of time available during visits to answer your questions. That's why today's dog owners educate themselves about canine needs and arrive at the veterinary office armed with information gathered from research on the Internet, other pet owners, magazines, and books—such as *Complete Care for Your Aging Dog*.

You are reading these pages because you cherish the relationship you share with your older dog—whether he's a mature seven-year-old or a teenage geriatric canine. *Complete Care for Your Aging Dog* offers not only great information about what physical and emotional changes may happen as your dog becomes a senior citizen, and how veterinary care can help; it also provides practical solutions to common problems, contact information for helpful products, educational and emotional support resources, and countless cost-saving home treatments.

Owners of aging dogs typically are willing to provide the extra care that keeps pets happy and comfortable. Medical help is a big part of that. Because many people are interested in alternative care in their own lives, a discussion of the pros and cons of "holistic" and conventional "allopathic" medicine for dogs is covered in the book. Both approaches offer great benefits for senior dogs, and combination therapies—called complementary medicine—may provide the greatest help.

On the conventional side, veterinary specialists such as surgeons and oncologists usually cost more, but they offer cutting-edge care that many dog owners are willing to fund in order to keep their dogs feeling good. In fact, the 2000–2001 survey by the American Animal Hospital Association (AAHA) indicates 74 percent of pet owners would go into debt for their pet's well-being. The cost of treatment is always a concern, though, so I've included sections titled "Bottom Line," which estimate how much a given diagnosis and therapy might cost.

More and more pet owners purchase health insurance for their dogs because it can make treatments and care for chronic illnesses—even cutting-edge and alternative therapies—quite affordable for the average owner. A checklist for evaluating pet insurance is included to help you make informed decisions. Another potential cost-saving measure is home nursing care that also can keep your dog happier and more comfortable during convalescence. The most common nursing techniques are described to help you decide which might be a good option for your situation.

Because of a lifetime of good care, many aging dogs stay healthy throughout their golden years and won't require anything but routine veterinary care. That makes it even more important for owners to know how to be good partners in their dog's good health. After all, you live with your dog all year long, you know him best, and you will be the first to recognize a problem and get help if something goes amiss.

Complete Care for Your Aging Dog offers practical ways to ensure a high level of enjoyment and happiness for both you and your dog as he continues to age. It's important to understand how bones and muscles change with age, and that aging eyes and ears can influence behavior, for example. Senior dogs often need more frequent bathroom breaks, and become less willing to walk up and down stairs. Providing a ramp or adding a doggy door keeps everyone happy and prevents "accidents" that upset human and dog alike. Many owners of aging dogs willingly rearrange their schedules to accommodate their pet—coming home for lunch provides an extra bathroom break for the dog, for instance. After all, it's what we do for our friends.

There are so many easy, simple, and inexpensive ways for you to keep an aging dog happy and healthy! This book provides guidelines to create your own "health report card" to keep track of normal versus warning signs, and learn when you can treat problems at home and when a veterinary visit is needed. It also includes all the latest research about how pet owners can maintain old-dog physical health by choosing the right nutrition, providing safe and effective exercise, using easy grooming tips, and making positive changes to the dog's home environment. Old dogs may lose their sense of smell, so that food is less appealing. Adding a bit of warm water may be all that's necessary to stimulate their flagging appetite.

As a dog ages, his social standing among the other pets in the household may change. That can be due to health issues, changes in his activity level, or reduced ability to hear and see. You can help him adjust to his new position and any physical limitations by using many of the tips offered in this book. Keeping the doggy soul healthy is equally important to quality of life, so you'll get ideas of ways to enrich your dog's emotional and mental health.

Throughout the book you'll find boxes with quick, helpful information to owners of aging dogs. For example, "Comfort Zone" offers product suggestions that are particularly applicable to the well-being of senior dogs. Look especially for "Golden Moments," heartwarming stories of real dogs and their people who are continuing to enjoy life while dealing with old-pet concerns. Read how Heidi regained her sight, how Green Machine still catches bad guys, and how Kramer continues to be an inspiration. If you're like me, you'll become a bit misty-eyed reading these inspirational stories that honor the love we share for our own dogs.

A frank discussion of quality-of-life issues—your own and the dog's—is also covered. Every pet partnership is different, and you have to be sensitive to your family and to your dog as to the best time to end his life. Grief is a normal part of losing a special dog. I've suggested ways to validate grief, help yourself and your children through this process, and honor the memory of a special pet.

Don't forget to take a look at the resources in the appendices, which include veterinary associations, subscription E-mail lists related to specific senior-dog concerns, and contact information for the products mentioned earlier in the book. There's also a list of must-have home remedies, a glossary of terms, and information about the experts who were interviewed for this book. You or your veterinarian can contact these experts through the university or clinic with which they're associated to see if your dog would benefit from their help.

I hope you'll find this book to be a valuable resource for senior-canine care that will benefit you, your dog, and your veterinarian. More than anything, *Complete Care for Your Aging Dog* is a celebration of the lifetime of love we share with our special pets. Today, pet owners have more and better options than ever before to ensure that they enjoy their dog's glorious golden years.

PART ONE

How Dogs Age

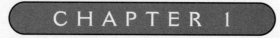

CHAPTER 1

Defining "Old"

What is considered "old" for a dog? The question is complicated, because it is determined by a combination of genetics, environment, and individual foibles. Consider human beings: one person may act, look and feel "old" at sixty-five, while another sixty-five-year-old remains an active athlete with a youthful attitude and appearance. The same is true for dogs. "Some dogs are old at six to seven years and some are old at ten to eleven years," says Steven E. Holmstrom, DVM, a veterinary dentist in San Carlos, California. The oldest dog on record was an Australian Cattle Dog who lived for twenty-nine years and five months.

A good definition of old age for an animal is the last 25 percent of its life span. Therefore if a dog lives to age sixteen, he'd be considered "old" at twelve years old, while a dog that lives only until age ten is considered old at seven-and-a-half.

Since we can't predict what an individual dog's life span will be, the beginning of old age is a bit arbitrary. Some generalities can be made based on a dog's size and known breed characteristics. Small dogs tend to live much longer than bigger dogs, and giant breeds definitely have a much shorter life span. In addition, certain "lines" of dogs may be longer lived than others, in the same way that some human families enjoy a much greater longevity than others. The life span of the parents and grandparents of your dog is a good predictor of how long you can expect your dog to live. People who share their lives with pedigreed canines have an advantage in that information about parentage can be tracked down through the dog's breeder.

Longevity of dogs having a mixed heritage are much more difficult to predict, even when they are the product of specific breeds. Despite claims that mutt dogs possess better health due to "hybrid vigor," these canines actually may inherit the very worst—or the very best—from their ancestors. Mixed-heritage dogs typically include two or more specific breeds in their family tree, and the fact that they were not carefully bred (so that "mixed" litters were prevented) may actually point to a poorer-than-average level of health for their parents.

Siblings within the same random-bred litter can vary greatly in size, behavior, and health, and it can be difficult (or even impossible) to find out an accurate history of the mixed-breed dog's ancestors. When all is said and done, one should expect mixed-breed animals to be neither more nor less healthy than their pedigreed ancestors—as long as they all receive the same level of care and attention.

The best predictor of longevity in mixed dogs, as in specific breeds, is the size of the pet. Generally speaking, the smaller the dog, the longer he will live.

Small dogs under twenty pounds—terriers, miniature Poodles, Lhasa Apsos, Shih Tzus, and the like—potentially have a life span of fifteen to seventeen years. Therefore, the onset of old age—when a pet becomes "senior"—would occur from about age eleven to thirteen for Toy breeds.

Medium to big dogs such as Labradors, German Shepherds, Rottweilers, and Golden Retrievers often live to age ten to twelve. They would therefore be considered old starting at about seven years.

Giant breeds (those weighing over eighty pounds or so) tend to become gray and show signs of age the earliest of all. Great Danes are considered old as early as five years and typically live for only seven to nine years. There certainly are exceptions to these generalities, with some very large dogs living healthy, comfortable lives well into their teen years.

To put this in perspective, consider that at age seven, a small-breed dog is equivalent to about forty-nine years in a human. A large-breed dog is the human equivalent of about sixty-five years, with giant breeds even older. To simplify matters, most veterinarians consider dogs to be "senior citizens" starting at about seven to eight years old, and to be geriatric at fourteen to fifteen.

Veterinarians used to concentrate their efforts on caring for young animals. Certainly, good care from the very beginning has a positive impact on how long and how well your dog will live. In the past, when pets began to develop age-related problems, people used to just get another pet. Today that attitude has changed, and both owners and veterinarians recognize that age is not a disease. Modern dogs age seven and older can still live full, happy, and healthy lives.

When physical and emotional changes do come with advancing age, they can often be managed successfully with very simple and inexpensive accommodations to the dog's environment. Today's owners are much more likely to treat senior and geriatric dogs than they would have in the past. "They want everything for that fifteen-year-old dog that you would do for a two-year-old dog," says Steven L. Marks, DVM, an internist at Louisiana State University. That benefits not only the animal, but also enriches and preserves the emotional bond owners have developed with their special dog during those seven, ten, sixteen or more years they've shared.

BENEFITS OF SENIOR PETS

Puppies go clear off the "cute factor" scale. However, they are works in progress, exciting yet difficult to predict, nonstop fun but also frequently frustrating. It requires much time, patience, and understanding to forge the kind of bond with puppies that we take for granted with our older canine friends.

Mature dogs have many advantages over puppies. Probably the biggest advantage is that together you have created a partnership, and already know each other and have adjusted to individual needs and foibles. All the hard work is done. She's been housetrained and tells you when she needs to "go"—and you know just how many hours you can be away from home before she's in dire straits. She's learned not to chew the TV remote control or your shoes, except for the old house slipper she's carried around like a teddy bear since you brought her home ten years ago. She reminds you when it's time for a pill and an afternoon nap—for both of you. And she acts like the new baby is her own pup, and showers the infant with attention, gentle play, and protective care—even putting up with toddler tail tugs with a patient doggy grin. Countless children have learned to walk while grasping the furry shoulder of a canine friend.

In fact, one of the best ways to introduce young children to the positive aspects of dogs is with a calm, temperament-sound adult animal. Parents already have their hands full dealing with infants and toddlers, and don't need the added stress of an in-your-face pup. Children can share birthdays with the aging dog and still be relatively young when the dog enters her golden years.

It's not unusual for young people to say that one special dog has *always* been a part of their life—and in times of family crises or emotional upset, the dog can ease the tension and help heal the pain simply by being there to pet and talk to. A broken heart, disagreements with siblings or parents, even physical or emotional trauma can all be helped by the mere presence of a dog that the child loves.

An older dog can be a stabilizing influence on children, teach responsibility and empathy for other living creatures, and even act as a social bridge toward making friends with their peers. For example, a child shy of interacting with other children because of a perceived disability often comes out of her shell when accompanied by a furry friend—the dog remains the focus of interaction rather than the child's "different" look or behavior. Older dogs often are ideal for such relationships, because they aren't as active as younger dogs, may be more patient, and have learned what to expect. There's a benefit to the old dog, too—playing and interacting with children keeps the doggy mind and body active and youthful.

The advantages of loving an older dog are not limited to children. Studies have shown that contact with dogs offers great physical and emotional health benefits to people, from children and adolescents to adults and senior citizens.

Couples whose children have left for college and are recent empty nesters can receive great comfort by the presence of a furry companion. People of any age who lose a spouse to divorce or death—but particularly older owners—benefit greatly from a dog's nonjudgmental love. For instance, petting a dog lowers the blood pressure, and caring for a dog gives owners a purpose to concentrate on beyond the hurt and pain. Going for walks, shopping for dog food, giving medicine to an old doggy friend, keeps people connected to the world and other people around them.

Old dogs are often the companions of aging owners because that old pet has the same problems they've got, says William Tranquilli, DVM, a professor and pain specialist at the University of Illinois. "They don't necessarily want a young pet. They want to do what they can to help their old buddy." They're willing to spend the money and often have more time to treat chronic disease to try to make the old animal more comfortable. And because the pets that we love are good for human health, just having a dog around can reduce the trips owners take to their own doctors. Some physicians recommend that heart attack survivors keep a pet, because it increases their survival.

People of all ages whose human family members live far away become even more emotionally dependent on the dog. In cases of elderly owners, Fritzie may be the only remaining family member they have. Of those pet owners who have a will, 27 percent have included provisions for their pets. Prolonging the dog's life touches on a host of social and emotional issues.

Dogs who have spent a decade or more with us have learned what we like and expect—and we've learned to anticipate the senior dog's needs, likes, and dislikes. Over the span of years, we build and then enjoy a comfortable companionship together. Our aging pets share with us our life experiences, successes and failures, joys and sorrows, and they represent milestones in our lives. They may have celebrated with us when we graduated school, married, and had children or grandchildren—or comforted us during convalescence, a lost job, or retirement. They have been there for us through everything. The more time we spend together, the greater our affection grows. Our compassion, love, and empathy for each other reach a depth that has no parallel in human existence.

"We share our secret souls with our pets in ways we wouldn't dare with another human being," says Dr. Wallace Sife, a psychologist and president of the Association for Pet Loss and Bereavement. "We're human beings, and love is love. Love for a pet is no different than love for another human being."

WHAT TO EXPECT

Pet owners relish spending time with their older dog. As she ages, the chances increase that she'll need more medical care. The most common health problems of senior dogs mirror those of aging humans, and include cancer, heart disease, arthritis, kidney failure, diabetes, obesity, and dental disease. Aging dogs are also prone to sensory loss; eyesight, hearing, and scent sense fade with age. A certain percentage of aging dogs also develop behavioral changes that mimic those of human Alzheimer's patients.

"People need to recognize that older animals get diseases more frequently, and most of these diseases are progressive," says Dr. Marks. Problems such as kidney or heart disease will not go away, but pets *can* live with these conditions and enjoy a good quality life for months to years after the diagnosis. Just how long treatment will help depends on the individual dog and the owner's commitment. "I don't think you can just say, 'This is a ten-year-old dog; let's call it quits,' " says Dr. Marks. "You have to look at it and say, 'This is a ten-year-old pet that has a disease. Let's see what we can do.' "

In fact, a large majority of old dogs remain relatively healthy throughout their golden years and won't require more than routine medical care. Some age-related conditions change only the dog's looks, and won't affect the way she acts or feels. For example, the fur on the ear fringes and the muzzle often turns gray, but dogs don't care about appearance. Another typical change turns the dog's eyes bluish or hazy because the lens loses flexibility, says Harriet Davidson, DVM, an ophthalmologist at Kansas State University. "It's the reason humans have to get glasses when they turn about forty," says Dr. Davidson, but dogs can't see up close anyway, so they don't even notice this normal aging change.

Even when they don't have special health care problems, though, all senior dogs require more emotional support and nutritional help than younger pets. As the most important person in your dog's life, it's up to you to help her make the transition into a graceful old age. Some changes will be minor and probably won't cause much of a change to your routine. Others may require bigger commitments on your part to help keep the dog happy and comfortable, as well as reduce the potential for aggravating age-related problems.

For example, you'll need to provide a new diet designed specifically for the needs of an older dog. If you have a food-motivated dog such as a Labrador, who eats anything that doesn't move faster than she does, the diet change won't be a hardship for either one of you. Dogs with more discriminating palates, though, may take a bit of adjustment to accept a new diet, particularly since their sense of smell and taste might interfere with how much they like it. You may need to adjust your schedule to increase meals from once or twice a day to three or four times to ensure she gets enough nutrition.

Similarly, some dogs will require more frequent bathroom breaks. That probably won't be a problem if she has a pet door, or spends much of her day in the yard. Otherwise, though, running home to let her outside over your lunch break may save your carpet and your relationship.

Something as simple as picking up her water bowl several hours in advance and giving her a last-minute pit stop prior to bedtime allows you both the luxury of sleeping through the night. Of course, it doesn't bother some folks to be cold-nosed awake at 3:00 A.M., particularly if you're getting up anyway for your own late-night potty break.

COMFORT ZONE: INDOOR BATHROOM ALTERNATIVES

You can teach old dogs new tricks, help out your pet, and make life simpler for yourself. Dogs that weigh thirty pounds or less can be trained to use a canine litter box or inside bathroom. That's very helpful for elderly owners, for those who live in cities or apartments far from the park, and for elderly or ill dogs who have less control or capacity to "hold" themselves for very long. Little dogs tend to hate going outside in cold weather, so an indoor alternative is particularly helpful. Dog litter is designed to be more absorbent to accommodate the greater urination needs (compared to cats), and also provides odor control. Larger particles won't track, and do not "clump," which can be a problem if dogs try to eat the material. Products currently available include:

- "Puppy Go Potty" (recycled paper fibers) made by Absorption Corp of California, can be purchased as a kit with all necessary supplies (including the litter box), training information, and both a phone and on-line "help" resource. More information is available at www.puppygopotty.com.
- "Secondnature" (a recycled-newspaper product) from Nestlé Purina PetProducts, comes with a training booklet in each bag of litter, and both a phone and on-line "help" resource. The company also markets specialized dog litter boxes in three sizes, which are usually larger than their feline counterparts, with one side cut away for easier access. More information is available at www.doglitter.com.
- "WizDog Housetraining Toilet" (http://wizdog.com/) is another alternative for indoor elimination, and costs about $30. It consists of a flat tray with a plastic grid that fits over the top, allowing canine feet to stay clean and dry as urine flows through to be caught by newspapers or an absorbent pad. It is designed for small to medium-size dogs, but units can be added to accommodate even large canines.

Aging dogs tend to lose stamina for the long walks and romps they enjoyed during their youth. Be aware that if you jog down to the corner store together, she may beg you to carry her back home—or take a long break to rest before starting back. She may also have trouble navigating stairs, getting into the car, or climbing onto a favorite sofa or the bed. Such dogs require a helpful boost up and down. You may need to find a more convenient place for her bed—one that's not elevated, for example, and is toasty warm from the morning sun. That can help relieve stiff joints.

If she's put on the pounds, as many dogs do when they get older, she

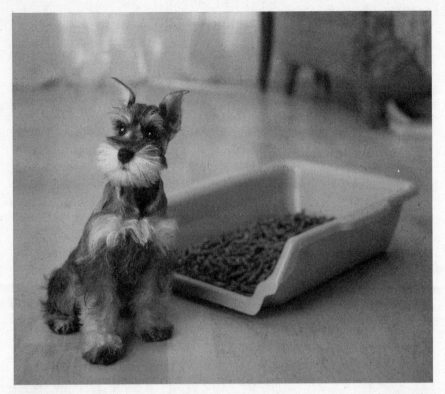

Canine litter products, such as Secondnature, can offer indoor bathroom facilities for aging dogs who have less ability to wait for potty breaks. *(Photo Credit: Second-nature dog litter/Nestlé Purina PetCare Company)*

shouldn't be left outside for long during hot weather. Overweight aging dogs overheat much more quickly and can have problems breathing and even die from temperature extremes. Cold weather poses the opposite problem when the skin and fur thins, and aging dogs become heat magnets during the winter months. Small dogs especially benefit from sweaters to ward off a chill, but old pets of any size relish a warm place to sleep and snuggle.

Although senior dogs are the same constant friend we've always known, they tend to become less patient as they get older. She'll rely more on routine, want her dinner *right now*, and demand to go outside *this instant*. She may continue to enjoy interaction with the other pets and children, but aging dogs tend to reach their tolerance level more quickly. Every dog is different, and adding a younger pet (or a new baby) to the household gives some dogs a kick in the tail like the fountain of youth. But others turn into canine curmudgeons if faced with any change in routine.

For instance, she may pine and be inconsolable should her favorite teenager leave for college, or a beloved companion dog dies. She could turn snippy if you shut her out of the new baby's room. At any age, and particularly as she grows older, it's important that the senior-citizen dog be made to feel she's still an important part of the family and included as much as possible. Instead of shutting the door to the nursery, put up a baby gate so she can watch and sniff and hear the new family member, and she'll be much more willing to take a positive interest.

Loss of hearing means previously well-trained dogs seem to ignore you. She may also startle more easily, so you'll need to explain to visitors and family members not to sneak up on her, or she might snap out of fear without meaning to. Some hearing-impaired dogs begin barking a lot more—they can't hear themselves, or you, and so use their "alarm cry" to get attention. Giving her extra treats or petting simply rewards the behavior and can make barking worse. Instead, a short "time-out" in a small room usually calms the barking, after which the quiet dog can rejoin the family. You'll also learn to stomp a foot, wave your hand, or use other visual signals to gain her attention. Dogs readily learn hand signals in lieu of voice commands, and adjust so quickly to dimming senses that you may not know anything is different at all.

If your dog loses her vision, you'll need to dog-proof the house to protect her from injury. Products designed for child safety can be adapted for use with elderly dogs. For example, a baby gate across the stairs will keep her from falling. Baby gates also work well to confine dogs into safe—or easily cleaned—areas of the home. "Safety Turtle" for pets (www.poolcenter.com) protects her from drowning should she fall into the swimming pool, leap out of a boat, or stumble into the lake. The Turtle band is attached to the dog's collar, the remote plugged into an outlet, and the alarm will sound if the Turtle band becomes submerged in water.

Some doggy day-care centers may make special arrangements for the needs of an older dog—for instance, ask about a private playtime where the ball is rolled on the ground rather than flipped through the air to be caught. They may partner her with dogs of similar size and age so as not to exhaust or overwhelm her. However, because aging dogs become so attuned to routine and familiarity, they often do better staying home with a visiting pet-sitter when you go out of town, rather than being boarded in a noisy, strange kennel.

If a dog requires special medications, you'll need to make arrangements with a person able to administer the treatment. Ask if one of the technicians at your veterinary clinic would be available. Other times, owners make the choice to postpone or forgo some trips in order to ensure that the needs of their dog—both physical and emotional—are met.

INSURANCE AND CARE PLANS

Although the cost for medical care for dogs is much less than comparable human treatments, paying for chronic care can be a financial burden for dedicated owners. In most cases, veterinarians are sympathetic and open to arranging payment plans when the cost exceeds your ability to pay.

Chronic care for aging dogs is one of the costliest periods for owners. Health care programs for animals provide older pets a better opportunity to get the service they need, by offering a way to pay a portion of the cost. Pet health insurance remains a relatively new concept.

Founded in 1980 with the support of 750 independent veterinarians, Veterinary Pet Insurance (VPI) is the oldest and to-date largest health insurance provider for dogs and cats. Since that date, a number of regional pet insurance companies have become available, but VPI is currently the only national provider of pet health insurance in the United States. "Likewise there is only one national provider in Canada, Pet Plan Insurance," says Randy Valpy, vice president and general manager of Pet Plan Insurance. "Both of our firms believe that the number of insured pets will grow fivefold during the next five years."

Today, the nation's estimated 23,000 veterinary hospitals each serve an average of twenty-five pet insurance policyholders, and that number continues to grow. "At VPI, we've grown 58 percent in the past five years," says Jack Stephens, DVM, founder of the company. He predicts that more pet owners will turn to insurance to take advantage of veterinary care that continues to rise in sophistication and cost. "We have, and always will, strive to make the miracles of veterinary medicine affordable," says Dr. Stephens.

Pet insurance typically works by reimbursing the dog owner for a predetermined amount that has been allotted for the specific veterinary service after it's been performed. For example, you would pay your veterinarian in full, then submit the receipts to the insurance company in order to receive payment back according to the amount designated in your dog's particular coverage schedule. "We don't tell the veterinarian what to charge," says Dr. Stephens. "But we do have a fee schedule so it controls our costs." VPI allows pet owners to choose their veterinarian.

Health programs like Pet Assure are not true insurance companies, and simply offer a percentage discount on any veterinary care across the board, regardless of health status, age, or preexisting condition. The Pet Assure service is limited to only those veterinarians enrolled in the program. Similarly, VetSmart Clinics (located across the country in many PETsMART stores) offer Banfield's Optimum Wellness Plans that discount many preventive care services to about 50 percent, with memberships that can be paid on a monthly basis. CareCredit, based in Anaheim, California, offers the clients of participating veterinarians the option of paying for expensive services on a monthly installment basis.

The amount covered varies from company to company, from plan to plan, and from city to city. Like human insurance, preexisting conditions may be disallowed, so you must buy the insurance before the dog develops the problem. Age also influences the cost.

VPI does not have a senior-pet policy, says Elizabeth Hodgkins, DVM, medical director and vice president of claims for VPI. "We will insure any pet, regardless of age. But premiums go up as the animal ages." For example, for about the same kind of coverage, a dog that's one year old will cost $200 a year, while an animal that's twelve costs about $400. "That's very similar to life insurance in people where you pay a whole lot more if you're fifty than if you're twenty," says Dr. Hodgkins.

A new program from PetCare Insurance recently introduced by Reader's Digest offers a policy specifically for older pets. QuickCare Senior is tailored coverage for accidents and illnesses common to older cats and dogs, including coverage for cancer, stroke, seizures, and heart problems. QuickCare Senior provides coverage for dogs over age eight. However, PetCare Insurance is not available in all states.

Companies also define the age breaks differently. For example, PetsHealthCare, based in Ohio, defines eligible dogs as being between the age of eight weeks and prior to turning nine, with additional premiums that apply to dogs over the age of nine; once the dog is enrolled, coverage can continue for the lifetime of your pet. For Pet Plan Insurance, the premiums stay the same as the dog ages, but the deductible increases for dogs at eight years and at eleven years of age for the basic plan. VPI defines age brackets for general premium increases as eight weeks to one year; one to four years; five to seven years; eight to nine years; and ten and over, with an increase each year thereafter.

It's important to purchase insurance as early as possible, before health problems develop. Not every preexisting condition disqualifies the dog from coverage—if he's fully recovered from being hit by a car, for example, that wouldn't preclude coverage. "But some pets become uninsurable as they get older," warns Dr. Hodgkins. "We will not insure pets that have already had cancer. If your pet has had a condition that is potentially life threatening and a recurrent problem, then it would become uninsurable."

In fact, some companies offer special coverage for catastrophic illness at a very low rate, if you purchase it when the dog is young and still healthy. VPI's "cancer rider" doubles the benefits for any diagnosis and treatment of cancer, and costs about $29 per year for a one-year-old dog compared to $120 per year for a twelve-year-old dog. The premium cost is locked in when it is purchased before the pet is two years old. "It's pennies a day," says Dr. Hodgkins. "You're going to spend way more on your Starbucks coffee than on the policy plus the cancer endorsement."

While VPI coverage is available nationwide, PetPlan Insurance is available only in Canada. PetsHealthCare Plan is available only in certain states. For instance, PetsHealthCare coverage is not offered in Montana, Idaho, Nevada, Wyoming, South Dakota, or Arkansas, although the company may expand to those states in the future. Some plans participate only with listed network veterinarians (similar to some human HMOs); others allow a choice of any practitioner. Additional differences may include variations in the cost of the deductible or higher premiums for particular dog breeds that may be predisposed to genetic health problems, or certain metropolitan areas that have higher typical veterinary fees.

Most basic plans will cover only accident and illness and routine care such as vaccinations, spay/neuter surgeries, teeth cleaning, and flea treatments. Other diseases generally require additional coverage. For example, VPI coverage addresses more than 6,400 health conditions, including diagnosis and treatment for liver, heart, and kidney disease, cataracts, diabetes, and cancer, which are most common in aging dogs.

Alternative medical care—chiropractic and acupuncture, for example— also may be covered as long as it is prescribed and performed by a veterinarian. Even experimental therapies such as kidney transplants, innovative cancer therapies, hearing aids, and the like may be covered when recommended by the veterinarian.

"We encourage specialists because we think specialists give the best treatment more quickly, which ultimately saves money in the end, and saves the animal," says Dr. Hodgkins. To encourage referrals to specialists, VPI policies start the benefit schedules over again when your dog is referred to a specialist. For example, if your veterinarian has performed $700 worth of the $800 treatment allotment, when you go to the specialist, you have that $800 available again.

In Canada the percentage of insured pets is only about 0.5 percent. "In Europe the acceptance of pet health insurance is far more common," says

Valpy. "In the U.K. over 15 percent of all pets are insured, and in Sweden over 41 percent of all pets are insured."

The numbers of insured pets in the United States barely doubles that of Canada. "We currently estimate that the entire pet health insurance industry is a little bit less than one percent of all pets owned in the U.S.," says Dr. Hodgkins. "Of that, not more than a third are seniors." That's unfortunate, she says, because older dogs stand to benefit the most from pet insurance. "You can have automobile insurance for forty years and never have an accident," says Dr. Hodgkins. "But sadly, your pet will ultimately sicken and die. Pet health insurance is something that, even if it takes ten or fifteen years for you to use it, you will."

SHOPPING FOR INSURANCE

A number of companies with different plans are available, and the ideal time to purchase coverage is when your older dog is still healthy. Ask these questions to help make the best choice for your individual situation:

1. Is your insurance offered in my state?
2. Are multiple plans available? Most companies have more than one level of coverage.
3. What are the eligibility requirements? Ask about dog age, preexisting conditions, and if veterinary records are needed in order to qualify (for dogs considered geriatric, records may be necessary).
4. When does coverage begin? There may be a thirty-day or longer "wait" period before illness coverage goes into effect. Also ask about any trial periods—some companies will refund your premium within a certain period if you're not satisfied.
5. How much is the annual premium? Ask about fee schedule coverage allowances for some of the most common senior pet conditions.
6. How much is the deductible? Is the deductible calculated on a per-year basis, or a per-incident basis?
7. Is there a price break to insure multiple pets?
8. Do you have any special "riders" for veterinary specialists, cancer coverage, or other senior-pet issues?
9. Is there a "maximum" benefit dollar amount? Is it calculated per year? Per diagnosis? Per lifetime?
10. Which breeds, if any, cost more to be covered? Are any breeds uninsurable?

Owners of aging dogs must make health care decisions that often are based on financial limitations. "There is nothing more frustrating for a veterinarian than knowing you can heal a sick patient, but the owner lacks financial resources and instructs you to put the pet down," says Dr. Stephens. Pet insurance may be an option that helps remove some of the burden and reduce what Dr. Stephens characterizes as "economic euthanasia."

Ask your veterinarian for a recommendation about pet insurance. You can also search the Internet. A brief list of contact information for representative companies is provided in Appendix A. Be aware that this industry is so new that companies may come and go, contact information may become outdated, and coverage could change.

"Get the insurance as soon as you can," advises Dr. Hodgkins. "Many older animals become ineligible because of the development of these diseases, and they're the same diseases that we'd happily pay for if they'd purchased the insurance before."

QUALITY OF LIFE

When we welcome our dogs into our hearts, we do so knowing they will not live as long as we'd like. That makes our time spent with them even sweeter. People who deeply love their dog have a strong commitment to keeping him not only healthy, but also happy during the golden years. With the advent of cutting-edge veterinary care, pets' lives can be extended longer than ever before.

However, a longer life isn't always a better life. "The quality of the patient's life is really our main concern and main business in veterinary medicine," says Laura Garret, DVM, an oncologist at Kansas State University.

What exactly is "quality of life"? Simply put, the term refers to the degree of comfort and enjoyment the pet experiences in day-to-day living. Measuring quality of life isn't always easy and depends a great deal on the individual animal, the owner, and the relationship they share. You know your dog best—what makes him happy, and how he acts when he feels good. So one of the best ways to look for answers is to compare your pet's attitude, activity level, and behavior when he's well to the way he is in the current situation.

For instance, do Fritzie's painful hips discourage him from walking—from even getting up at all—when he used to dance with delight at the mere word? Does Fluffy hide when medication time rolls around, even though she used to run to you at any excuse? Does Jazzie refuse to eat, even though his life's passion used to be the food bowl? Does Jeep no longer recognize you at all? Quality of life means your senior pet feels good, stays connected with you, and enjoys his remaining time in familiar, safe, and loving surroundings.

The right treatment can make an incredible difference. Because chronic problems such as painful arthritis or vision loss develop gradually, pet owners often don't recognize them until symptoms become severe. At that point, Fritzie's new behaviors may be attributed to "old age" when in fact treatments can turn back the clock and return him to the activities of a younger pet. Pain medication likely won't prompt leaps out of old Fritzie, but it can put him back on his feet for happy walks with his favorite people.

Remember: old age is *not* a disease. Don't assume you must accept these changes of behavior just because your dog has reached seven years old or more.

TREATMENT ADVICE

It's important to have realistic goals. While a cure isn't always possible, health conditions of older dogs can often be controlled to ensure a good quality of life. Your veterinarian can help you decide on the best choices based on your dog's situation, your own emotional and financial circumstances, and your "comfort level" regarding home care.

Often people are much more capable of handling home care than they think. The turning point may come, for example, when you realize that giving an insulin injection can save your dog's life. But dealing with your emotions upon learning that your dog has cancer can be difficult, because we bring our own fears to the situation. Your veterinarian can help explain what to expect in the way of prognosis, treatment, and any side effects. In many cases the situation isn't as bad as we fear. The dog with painful bone cancer may, in fact, welcome amputation that takes the pain away. He doesn't worry about other dogs looking at him "funny" and is just delighted to feel good again.

Talk with your veterinarian and other family members not only to make informed decisions, but also to reduce any guilty feelings down the road, says Barbara Kitchell, DVM, an oncologist at the University of Illinois. "Some people are really haunted by those kinds of decisions," she says.

Ask yourself, Are you the kind of person who will forever say, "I should have . . ."? Or are you the kind of person who makes choices, goes through with therapy, and accepts the outcome knowing everyone has tried their best? "That critical decision-making period with the client is not an irrevocable decision either," says Dr. Kitchell. "We start down the road, and if you feel the quality of life is not what you want, we change course. We can stop at any time."

There are often financial considerations. Certain therapies are more expensive than others, and not all are affordable for everyone. Even when the optimum therapy is cost-prohibitive, other more economical options may be available. For example, although a $3000 hip-replacement surgery may be the ideal solution for an arthritic dog, less expensive surgeries are also available and offer good results. Or perhaps pain medication offers the best choice to manage the condition. Similarly, there's a huge range of chemotherapy drugs available. "There's a menu of options you can select for that individual client's needs," says Dr. Kitchell. Each animal is so different that it's impossible to predict which choice—the most expensive or the most economical—will produce the best results. "I want to give you good quality time with this animal, and nobody can predict how much time that will be," she says.

"I get a lot of joy out of being able to help that animal do really well throughout the rest of its geriatric life," says Signe Beebe, DVM, a veterinary acupuncturist and herbal specialist. When holistic treatment is combined with mainstream "Western" medicine, she says the dog is more likely to remain vital and enjoy life up until the very end—rather than experiencing a traumatic decline with intermittent hospitalizations. "My clients want to try everything they can to have a good quality of life for their animal. And when they can no longer have that good quality of life, then it's time for that animal to pass on," says Dr. Beebe.

We know that our dogs won't live forever. Dogs don't know that, though. Tomorrow doesn't exist for them. They don't know or care—or worry—about what happens in an hour, a week, or a month. Dogs live in the "now." And that frees them to greet you each day with joyful, innocent abandon.

Dogs provided with good care during the course of a terminal illness die with a lot of dignity and tremendous grace, says Dr. Kitchell. "Death is a process. And you see an animal go through that process. They say, 'I love you. But it's time for me to go.' You see them get themselves ready," she says. "It's so beautiful to watch it, and it's so beautiful to be with them, and there's so much peace at the end of it that it's a lovely thing."

Four out of ten dogs and cats are aged seven years and older. This aging population constitutes more than 50 percent of patients seen by veterinarians—44.8 million pets—according to surveys by the American Veterinary Medical Association and others. The numbers will climb as loving owners continue to provide the best care possible for their aging dogs.

Golden Moments: Collie Love

Anne Ewing Rassios, an American geophysicist making her home in Grevena, Greece, says she and her husband Adamos have always had several dogs. Most live out at the family workshop, where their duties include guarding the property from not only human predators, but also from wolves or bears that wander down from the nearby Pindos and Mt. Olympus mountains. Several years ago, when the family decided to get a dog specifically to "keep our son, Mike, in line," says Anne, they discovered Collie love.

A couple Anne met at work offered her the choice of a pup. "I look in the eyes for a *spark*," she says. "Doing that, we've always managed to have dogs that are far too intelligent for their own good. Scottsie had the *spark*."

She brought the male cinnamon-and-white Scottish Collie home, planning that he'd live with the other dogs out at the workshop. But Scottsie wasn't like any dog they'd ever had before. "He became ill, wouldn't eat," she says, and the humans pined for him, too, so they raised Scottsie in their home.

It wasn't long before everyone in the village began to recognize the beautiful

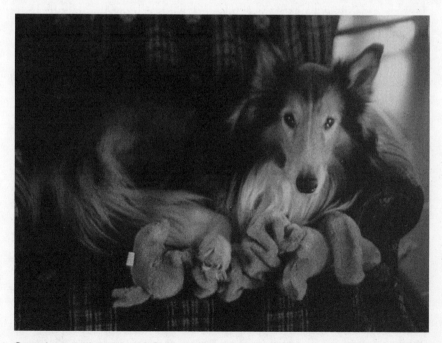

Scottsie, a twelve-year-old Collie, is enjoying his golden years in Greece. *(Photo Credit: Annie Rassios)*

dog. Anne says he learned to also answer to "Lassie" so the children who greeted him on the street wouldn't be disappointed. "He has a whole repertoire of tricks to do for little children—who are convinced he really *is* Lassie—and he can fetch any of his toys by its name," she says. "So why couldn't we teach him, 'Scottsie, where are the car keys?' 'Scottsie, where's the remote control?' 'Where's Daddy's cell phone, Scottsie?' We really missed an opportunity!"

Walks in the woods have kept him happy, active, and healthy for more than a decade, and he adores his job on pigeon patrol. "We're up in a penthouse here, with an enormous 1,100-square-foot balcony around the house—and we're en route for pigeon central." Scottsie delights in herding the pigeons away to keep the balcony clear of pigeon droppings.

"He has a thing for tortoises. He can't hurt them, so I let him bark and scratch for about ten minutes while I pretend he isn't my dog," says Anne. "I walk off; eventually he realizes I'm gone and races to find me." She says he also has a "thing" about men with beards. "He's been known to growl at visiting Greek priests here to bless the building, but welcome the smooth-shaven Jehovah's Witnesses with bounds and leaps of undying affection."

Scottsie is a dog very in tune with the people he loves, and gives and demands affection with equal enthusiasm. "He'll place his rump under your hand for a scratch if you're not paying attention," says Anne, "and he helps around the house by waking up Adamos on command—he digs through blankets to find him." He also has a peculiar talent for knowing who is on the phone when it rings. "I have no idea how he does it, but if it's from my Mom, our son Mike, or a friend, Scottsie goes wild with joy, barking and dancing. If it's a stranger, a wrong number, or someone selling something, he doesn't even wake up."

Since their son Mike left two years ago for college in the States, Scottsie has missed him awfully, says Anne. "Scottsie is twelve years old. We've denied the significance of the graying nose for several years, because his health and energy have been excellent." But he has finally become noticeably stiff in the back legs, his gait has changed, and he "misses" his jumps onto the couch from time to time. "We help him up to the couch when he gets stuck halfway," she says. "And we have started to include him in our yearly visits to the Aegean, because, though he hates to swim, taking him out and making him swim seems to be really good for him."

He let some other dogs browbeat him into a tummy-up defense earlier this year, and Anne says this loss of status seems to have affected him emotionally. "He definitely is no longer the alpha male of the group, and defers to the pack."

More recently, Scottsie developed an eye problem that cortisone and antibiotics haven't helped. "It doesn't seem to bother him, though." The vet says an operation at the vet school in Thessaloniki could help, but anesthesia risk would be worse for him than the eye problem.

"Meanwhile he's a sweeter dog than ever, and we are loving him more than ever," says Anne. "We all know what's coming up and are enjoying each other as much as we can."

She concludes that only families who are willing to devote time and love will do well with a Collie. "Collies require a special emotional commitment. Collies have to be with families," says Anne. "They aren't dogs; they are family."

CHAPTER 2

The Aging Process

Aging is a natural process. Early in life as the puppy grows, her body builds new tissue, repairs injuries, and maintains multiple functions that allow her to thrive in harmony with the world around her. Growth slows and stops once adulthood is reached, but at the microscopic level, nothing is static. Cells are continuously created, function for a short time, then die and are replaced. Systems such as the kidneys have built-in redundancies and reserves that allow the healthy dog to adapt to internal physical stresses as well as to influences from the environment.

On its most basic level, the progression of age interferes with the ability of the body to bounce back. Normal reserves are depleted when cell turnover—the ability of the body to create new cells—slows down or stops altogether. Aging dogs lose the ability to self-repair, protect, and maintain good health. They become more vulnerable to injury and illness, and take much longer to recover.

Eventually, old organ systems are unable to keep up with normal demands. There may be a drop in the production of certain hormones responsible for regulating critical functions of the body. All this has a cascade effect on other parts of the body. For instance, lungs unable to fuel the body with sufficient oxygen cripple the ability of the liver to do its job, and that in turn poisons the dog when her liver can't detoxify waste products.

The aging process is not fully understood, but one theory suggests that the body is genetically programmed to live only a certain length of time, and that the brain automatically hits the off switch when it reaches that point. Another theory maintains that cells can replicate—reproduce themselves—only a certain number of times before they lose the ability. This genetic aging is dictated by the dog's breed and inherited tendencies from her family line. Just as some human families live longer, some dog families are longer-lived than others.

Biological rust, more technically called oxidation, is a normal part of living. Just as metal rusts when exposed to air, foods spoil and fats turn rancid after long-term exposure to oxygen. The body's cells are also bathed in oxygen, which is necessary for many normal functions. But prolonged exposure to oxidation causes dogs to age at an accelerated rate and develop disease.

Mitochondria, tiny organlike structures inside each cell that are rich in fats, proteins, and enzymes, produce energy for the cell through respiration. This process not only generates energy, but also creates highly unstable and reactive molecules called free radicals. Oxidation in living tissue results when free radicals try to combine with normal molecules of the cells. This damages the cell walls and DNA, causing disease and accelerated aging.

"The nervous system tissue is especially vulnerable to attack by free radicals," says Blake Hawley, DVM, a veterinarian with Hill's Pet Nutrition. "An aged mitochondrion produces less energy but produces more of these toxic free radicals, so it's really important that as the cell ages, we find ways to absorb or attack those free radicals that are produced."

Other influences outside of genetics also speed up the aging process. For example, environmental factors include damage from ultraviolet light, or toxins in the air, water, or food. Injury, such as a fracture, speeds up the age-related joint degeneration known as arthritis. Proper nutrition sustains cell regeneration, while deficiencies in nutrition interfere with this process. Emotional stress suppresses the immune system and allows damage from parasite or viral infections, which can irreparably damage the body and contribute to accelerated aging.

Most dogs begin to slow down by the time they reach seven years or so. These changes are very gradual and subtle, though, and often we don't notice any significant changes. Even the veterinarian may not detect signs of aging without special tests, until they become obvious, at which point the damage may already be irreversible.

HOW AGE AFFECTS THE BODY

Age affects different parts of the body in different ways. Changes in one body system often interact with, and prompt changes in, other systems as well. For instance, painful joints that keep your dog from exercising can prompt weight gain, which makes it even more painful to move. The resulting obesity increases the chance of diabetes, and complications from diabetes may cause cataracts that result in blindness.

Cancer is another example. Aged dogs are most commonly affected by tumors when the normal age-related breakdown in the cell-replication system becomes abnormal. The mutant cancer cells can spread and affect multiple body systems, and sometimes mimic symptoms of other age-related conditions. Bone cancer of the leg, for example, causes pain and limping similar to arthritis.

It's important to understand how age affects the different body systems so you are alert to subtle changes in your dog that may point to serious problems. Catching problems early is the best way we have of successfully treating them, and keeping your dog happy and healthy.

The Senses

Dogs are above all sensory creatures. They learn about the world around them, and interact with humans via their five senses: touch, taste, scent, sight, and sound. In fact, dogs are blessed with sensory abilities above and beyond those their owners enjoy. They rely on hearing and scent, in particular, to a much greater degree than people do.

A lifetime of use and insult from their environment often causes damage to the sensory organs, which means they dim over time. And as with humans, there are normal age-related changes to the senses that every older dog will develop if he lives long enough. As far as we can tell, though, the dog's enjoyment of touch sensation—petting, snuggling, and contact with beloved owners—does not dim with age.

"All dogs get visual impairment, and all dogs get hearing impairment," says Benjamin Hart, DVM, a veterinary behaviorist at the University of California—Davis. Certainly that affects their behavior. What's important, though, is that sensory loss usually bothers owners much more than it bothers the pet. Dogs have an incredible ability to compensate by using their other senses, so we often don't recognize that there's an impairment until very late in the game.

Aging Eyes

Lawrence Myers, DVM, a professor of anatomy at Auburn University, developed a testing technique to measure how well dogs can see. "Visual acuity in the dog is fairly close to that of the human, probably a little less," he says. That's why dogs of any age may have trouble seeing the last bit of food in the bowl—they can't focus well at that distance."

Normal canine vision changes are similar to those of their owners. For example, people over the age of forty often need reading glasses to see close objects. This age-related vision change, called presbyopia, also affects dogs. It's caused by a normal change called nuclear sclerosis that causes the lens in the eye to turn hazy, inflexible, and less able to focus on close objects. "It still allows light and vision to go through," says Paul A. Gerding, Jr., DVM, an ophthalmologist at the University of Illinois. "That should be differentiated from cataract development."

The most common eye problems pet owners would notice in aging dogs are dry eye and cataracts. "Cataracts occur at all ages, but there's more likelihood as an animal ages, just as a person, that cataracts develop," says Dr. Gerding. Cataracts develop when the lens of the eye turns white and opaque, so the dog loses her vision.

In certain breeds, tear production can decrease with age and results in a condition called dry eye. When not enough tears are produced, the lack of lubrication prompts painful inflammation and/or damage to the cornea when the eye dries out. Also, dogs that have prominent eyes such as Pekingese are more prone to eye damage that may interfere with tear production and result in painful dry-eye conditions.

Glaucoma is another eye problem more typical of older dogs. It is extremely painful and, as with cataracts, can result in blindness. Loss of sight won't stop your dog from being a good pet, though. Vision-impaired and blind dogs tend to rely more on their other senses, such as hearing, as well as memory of certain landmarks to get around safely. Therefore, keeping the furniture in the same location becomes very important for blind dogs, says Dr. Myers.

Aging Ears

Although there's no particular breed predisposition to age-related hearing loss, dogs that hunt and are exposed to very loud noises like gunshots for years and years are more prone to ear damage. Even without damage,

age-related hearing loss, termed presbycusis, shows up in any animal if it lives long enough, says George M. Strain, DVM, a professor of neuroscience at Louisiana State University. Hearing loss can't be reliably predicted, but once it occurs, it continues to get worse with time.

Dogs can't tell us they're hard of hearing, and many hide it from their people. "They compensate by paying more attention to their other senses, so they may become more visually attentive, pay attention to vibration cues, air current, and things like that," says Dr. Strain. "Owners generally are unaware this is happening until it reaches a critical point where the animals can't cope very well—the dog doesn't come when they call, or startles easily."

Aging Taste

Changes in flavor perception are thought to reflect those experienced by aging humans, says Nancy E. Rawson, Ph.D., of the Monel Chemical Senses Center, a nonprofit research institute in Philadelphia dedicated to research in the fields of taste, smell, chemical irritation, and nutrition. "Young dogs apparently use taste very little in expressing food preferences, but it is possible that as olfaction [sense of smell] wanes with age, taste becomes more important," says Dr. Rawson.

The taste system of dogs is used as a model for people because they are so similar. Interestingly, the dog's taste receptors don't stop in the mouth, but extend down into the larynx. Dogs can taste and seem to prefer a "sweet" taste, from both carbohydrates and meaty sources, and salty flavors, and neither seems to be affected by age. Sour perception and bitter tastes are more sensitive to aging changes.

Chemical irritations and "mouth feel" influence how well the dog likes or dislikes a flavor. These can be influenced by changes in saliva content, for example, caused by dehydration that commonly develops in aged dogs. Disease or medication can reduce or increase the sensitivity of the mouth and tongue, and alterations in taste (and smell) can remain even after the disease is cured and the medicine is stopped. Dental disease may create a hypersensitive mouth, interfere with chewing ability, and produce unpleasant tastes and odors that prompt the dog to refuse certain foods.

Warming foods increases the volatility of tastes and scents to make them more intense and appealing to the aging dog's palate. Antioxidants may hold promise for prevention of age-related scent and taste loss, says Dr. Rawson.

Aging Nose

Scenting ability is arguably the most important sense for dogs, but few studies have documented exactly what happens to scenting acuity in relation to age. Nor do we know how much less acute a dog's sense of smell becomes, or whether the loss is due merely to age or to environmental factors as well.

"It can be a fairly mild sort of injury," says Dr. Myers. "I warn dog handlers and trainers not to rap across the muzzle because you have some risk of damage to the turbinate bones, which contain the olfactory mucosa, the receptor sheet for the olfactory portion of the system." This region can also be damaged by a number of respiratory diseases such as canine parainfluenza and distemper—even subclinical cases where there are no signs of illness—and endocrine diseases including hypothyroidism, Cushing's disease, and diabetes. Periodontal disease can also produce unpleasant odors that interfere with scenting ability.

Age-related losses in the sense of smell result from changes in the anatomy—scent cells aren't replaced as often—and at the molecular level when existing nerve cells and "messenger" molecules in the nose become less sensitive. Reduce salivation or altered nasal mucus composition can also impact the way odor chemicals are dissolved and detected, says Dr. Rawson.

"There tends to be a significant drop off in olfactory acuity in dogs at about ten years of age," says Dr. Myers. This loss may be especially hard on working dogs used in scent detection. Scenting ability of police "mantrailers" used to find lost children or Alzheimer's patients, and the bomb- and arson-detection dogs, can be a matter of life and death. The weekend hunter's companion dogs, and service dogs partnered with wheelchair-bound people, also rely on scent detection to find and retrieve the right object. Your dog may have trouble finding her favorite toy or treat once scenting ability fades.

Pet dogs may not suffer a great hardship from losing their sense of smell. "That's a very subjective sort of thing," says Dr. Myers, "but I certainly think there is some loss of quality of life."

Dr. Rawson says that as the dog ages, the scent-receptive cells become "more broadly tuned," and less able to discriminate between subtle differences between odors. "Reduced ability to detect the aroma of food can also cause a particular taste to seem more intense," she says, citing similar experiences with aging people who frequently complain that food tastes too salty. "Food selection tends to become less varied with age, and this may relate to a tendency to self-select those items that continue to be perceived as intensely as in youth, such as sweets," says Dr. Rawson. As a result, food flavor perception and preference may change as the dog ages.

Golden Moments: Led by the Nose

Ellen Ponall met her dog, Sherlock Tracers Starlight, more than nine years ago. "I've bred and trained Bloodhounds since 1972, and he got his call name because I color-code my dogs when they're born," she says. His birth order just happened to give him a green neck ribbon. He's been Green Machine ever since.

When Ellen retired as a senior service officer with the Glendale Heights Police Department, she and Green didn't stop working. "I got real involved

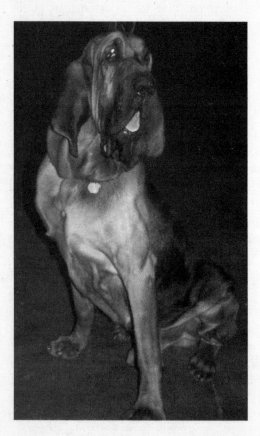

This nine-year-old Bloodhound, Green Machine, hasn't slowed down and continues to work in search and rescue. *(Photo Credit: Amy D. Shojai)*

with North American Search Dog Network, and am still on call by the police department."

Now nine years old, Green's scenting ability has only gotten better with age. "He's still my main man," says Ellen. She calls him the biggest mush in the world—the 112-pound Bloodhound once tried to crawl into her lap when he thought a hedgehog at a Humane Society event would eat him alive! But he's a whole different dog when the harness goes on. Says Ellen, "Green gets very upset if the younger dogs take his place—all the major cases are still his."

Recently, Ellen and Green were called out in the middle of a foggy night to find a gentleman suffering from Alzheimer's who had wandered away from home. Ellen was told the person couldn't go farther than a block because of his health limitations. "But Alzheimer's people don't realize they're old, and they have more stamina and oomph than the families give them credit for. They always go farther than you expect," says Ellen.

Green took a good whiff of the man's scent, and they were off and running after his trail. "When he's working, man, he moves! He really pulls, and you're not going to stop him," says Ellen. The police officers on the case didn't know Ellen or have any confidence in her dog when Green led them much farther than the family thought the missing man could go.

Suddenly the dog's head went up, and Ellen knew they'd found the man. "We crossed the street and Green zoomed in between two trailers to a little old man standing there." The dog is trained to do a "stand-up ID," which means he jumps up on the person and gives big kisses. "The little gentleman said, 'Where were you? I've been looking all over for you!' "

Ellen says it's exciting and satisfying to get the bad guys off the street, but it's even more rewarding to find lost people and especially children.

Ellen currently has twelve dogs in her household, and routinely works with older animals. "Veronica was thirteen, totally blind and still working. They don't need their eyes. It didn't bother her nose a bit," says Ellen. Green's nine-year-old sister, Purple, still begs to work but isn't as active anymore. "She has cancer, so I'm choosing not to work her," says Ellen. "She's doing well, she's not in any pain, and she's bouncing around. She's a happy camper." Ellen's fifteen-year-old Basset Hound doesn't really count as a working dog, but he thinks he's a Bloodhound, and he keeps up with the youngsters.

Ellen credits her dogs' working longevity to good conditioning and an excellent rapport with her veterinarian. She also relies on intuition and the close bond she shares with her dogs. "I'm constantly touching them, feeling lumpy-bumpies; that's a daily check. And exercise is key to keeping these guys in good health." Besides regular training work, all of her dogs have their own swimming pools. She keeps them lean because they work and feel better.

Ellen admits that age has changed Green. In his youth he'd chew through walls and kennels to get to the girl dogs. "He's mellowed; he's become more solid," she says. "All the changes have been positive ones."

Ellen knows that Green's career as a search-and-rescue dog may be nearing its end. "I don't like to think about it," she says. As long as his health remains good, and he loves the work, Green Machine will continue to do what he was born to do—with lots of big kisses along the way.

Bones and Muscles

By the time a dog becomes a senior citizen, her bones have begun to lose density and become weaker and more brittle. "We expect dogs at seven to eight to heal more slowly from a fracture," says James L. Cook, DVM, an orthopedic surgeon at the University of Missouri. "That's when we start to see a lot of the manifestations from arthritis in respect to the joints." Slowed healing and bone loss are likely due to the body's decreased capacity to regenerate bone cells. The cartilage wears thinner and becomes more brittle over time, and the ligaments and tendons connecting the joints sometimes stretch, become less flexible, and tear more easily. Arthritis in multiple joints becomes much more prevalent.

Muscles become less able to use nutrition efficiently. Dogs tend to slow down as they age, and a reduction in exercise prompts a gradual loss of not only muscle mass but also of bone density.

"Muscle mass is an extremely important metabolic reservoir," says Dan Carey, DVM, a veterinarian with the Iams Company. The body uses muscle as an energy source during illness or other debilitation. Human studies show that ill people with reduced muscle mass don't survive as well as those with healthy muscle mass, says Dr. Carey. Muscle mass is important in a dog's survival as well.

Digestion

The digestive system includes the mouth, teeth, stomach, intestines, pancreas, and liver. Digestion involves processing nutrition and eliminating waste. One of the greatest digestion-related problems of aging dogs is obesity, or "overnutrition." The dog's metabolism slows until her caloric requirements decrease by 20 to 40 percent during the last one-third of her life. Older dogs may continue to eat as much as they did when younger, but they don't burn nearly as many calories. And certain types of dogs, primarily the giant breeds such as Great Danes, which have large, deep chests, become more prone to gastric dilatation-volvulus (bloat) the longer they live, says Colin Burrows, BvetMed, a surgeon and internist at the University of Florida. Bloat is characterized by the deadly distension and twisting of the stomach.

Aging Teeth

Dogs are incredibly mouth-oriented. They use their mouths and teeth the way we use our hands, to carry objects and investigate their world. They also simply enjoy mouthing and chewing things. Over a lifetime of use, dogs often simply wear down or even break teeth as a result of recreational chewing.

Besides mechanical damage, tartar and plaque buildup cause dental disease that can ultimately result in loss of teeth and also impact the health of the rest of the body. "Having periodontal disease is analogous to having an open wound," says Bill Gengler, DVM, a veterinary dentist at the University of Wisconsin. Oftentimes the gum tissue is no longer attached to the tooth, and the root and bone are exposed, allowing bacteria to invade the circulating bloodstream. When an animal chews, she disturbs diseased gums and teeth enough to cause bacterial showering, says Dr. Gengler. The bacteria float along in the blood, then get stuck—filtered out—when the passages grow narrow. The bacteria are predominantly filtered out in the capillary beds of the liver and the kidneys, and can damage these organs. When this bacteria-laden blood passes through the valves of the heart, it can also cause endocardiosis, says Dr. Gengler. Endocardiosis is a thickening of the heart valves that leads to congestive heart failure and is a common cause of heart disease in the dog.

In addition to other mouth changes, the dog's sense of taste and salivary production decrease. That can have an impact on the dog's appetite and what she wants to eat.

Aging Stomach and Intestines

"The gastrointestinal tract in dogs is relatively well protected from the ravages of time," says Dr. Burrows. Some older people tend to lose a little bit of their digestive capacity, but that doesn't appear to be a significant problem for dogs. "Healthy geriatric dogs have perfectly normal digestion," agrees Dottie LaFlamme, DVM, a veterinary nutritionist at Nestlé Purina.

However, unhealthy animals may be less metabolically efficient as they age. There's evidence that some older dogs can digest the protein just as well, but they may not be as able to turn it into fuel. "Older dogs also need more protein than young-adult dogs to help maintain the protein reserves," says Dr. LaFlamme. Among other things, protein allows the immune system to work optimally, and protein also maintains muscle strength.

As dogs age, the normal bacterial population in their intestinal tract starts to increase in numbers. The most common type of bacteria can cause diarrhea when the organism penetrates and colonizes the lining of the intestine, says Dr. Carey. "Other types of bacteria actually secrete their own toxin," he says. They don't have to invade tissue—just the presence of this toxin can cause intestinal inflammation and other problems.

Older animals are much more likely to develop other diseases that may cause secondary changes in digestion. For example, aging dogs are much more prone to ulcers that develop as a result of metabolic and endocrine diseases such as kidney disease and Cushing's disease, or as a side effect of some oral medications used to manage arthritis pain.

Chronic constipation or diarrhea are not specifically "old dog" conditions, but they may affect geriatric pets. Obesity and lack of exercise can contribute to constipation, as can a decrease in the ability of the intestines to move waste along. The most common cause of colitis (inflammation of the colon) is improper diet, such as fatty table scraps. Stress can lead to bacterial overgrowth within the colon. For a dog with colitis, "fat restriction may be beneficial because fat absorption and digestion depends on enzymes that are found in the very tip of the villi that line the intestine, and this is the area that's damaged first," says Dr. LaFlamme.

Aging Pancreas and Liver

The pancreas produces enzymes that are vital to digestion, and both the production of gastric and pancreatic secretions decrease as the dog ages. Similarly, the enzymes produced by the liver for metabolizing nutrients and detoxifying the body decline with age. These organs continue to function well, though, even when they're not at 100 percent capacity.

When dogs require one or more medications, and the liver is functioning at less than full capacity, there may be trouble. "You need to be a little more cautious about medications with older animals," says Cynthia R. Leveille-Webster, DVM, an internist at Tufts University. "Old pets are often on multiple medications, and drug interactions can affect how they are handled by the liver." For instance, certain drugs can inhibit the normal production of liver enzymes. Therefore, if the liver is functioning at 70 percent and doing well, but a drug reduces that to 35 percent, the body will suffer the consequences. Among other things, reduced efficiency compromises the liver's ability to metabolize medications properly.

Endocrine System—Hormones

The endocrine system, which controls a dog's metabolism, includes the hormone-producing glands: pituitary, thyroid, parathyroid, pancreas, adrenals, ovaries, and testes. Hormones are a kind of "messenger" molecule secreted by endocrine glands and carried by the bloodstream to various distant body sites, with instructions to alter that target tissue's function. Hormones may speed up or slow down digestion, for instance, or regulate the female's estrus cycle.

Hormones, made either of protein or a type of specialized fatty substance called a steroid, regulate body functions and coordinate interactions between the different body systems. Too much or too little of a given hormone can cause disease. For example, not enough insulin results in diabetes, and too much testosterone can cause a perianal (near the anus) tumor to grow.

In particular, hormones produced by the thymus, thyroid, testes, and ovaries decrease as the dog ages. Dogs that have been neutered and had their testes and ovaries removed won't be affected, but the estrus cycle and libido of breeding animals may wane or be disrupted. If thyroid function falls off too far, hypothyroidism may result. Other hormone imbalances may cause a variety of skin changes, such as hair loss, thinning or thickening of the skin, or even color changes.

Older dogs slow down in part because their metabolic rate goes down, says Dr. LaFlamme. "There's less activity, so they're burning fewer calories. That can induce or worsen obesity," she says. Obesity, the most common nutritional disease of dogs, rarely is a product of diet alone—hormones often are intimately involved. For example, obesity can be a consequence of hypothyroidism, or a precursor of diabetes when fat suppresses the action of the hormone insulin.

Hormone imbalances become more common as the dog ages because of normal wear and tear on the organs, and also because age-related diseases like cancer often target the endocrine system. The pituitary gland pretty much rules how the rest of the endocrine system works, so anything that interferes with this "master gland" can potentially wreak havoc all over the body.

The most common age-related endocrine disorders include Cushing's disease, in which the adrenal gland secretes an excess of cortisol; and diabetes mellitus, an inability of the body to produce and/or use insulin. Both diseases are discussed in further detail later in the book. Problems like hypothyroidism (a greatly slowed metabolism prompted by the diseased thyroid) and Addison's disease (the opposite of Cushing's, not enough steroids produced by adrenals) are not considered typical "old dog" diseases. They can affect seniors, but most typically they first develop before the onset of old age.

Heart and Lungs

The cardiovascular system includes the heart, blood, and lymph, and functions to transport oxygen and nutrients to, and carry waste products from, all parts of the body. In older dogs, fluid retention (edema) can be prompted by tumors or other disorders that block the normal flow of the lymphatic vessels. Old-dog diseases such as kidney or liver disease may predispose the dog to bleeding disorders, or even cause a reduction in the production of blood. Anemia is a reduction in the number of circulating red blood cells, and ultimately reduces the amount of oxygen available to the body.

Heart attacks and arteriosclerosis are rare, but dogs can be born with heart abnormalities—congenital defects such as a hole in the heart or valve problems. Acquired heart disease and heart failure are among the most common diseases affecting older dogs, and develop over time. With age, the overall weight of the dog's heart increases while pumping efficiency decreases, and the walls of the large arteries in the body become thicker and less flexible. Basically, it becomes harder for the heart to work efficiently.

Acquired valvular disease is the leading cause of heart disease in dogs and is considered a disease of old age. About one third of all dogs over the age of twelve are affected when the heart valves simply start to wear out. It's most common in smaller breeds. Heart failure results when the damaged muscle is no longer able to move blood throughout the body properly.

The respiratory system is composed of the nose, larynx, trachea, bronchial passages, and lungs. This delivery system supplies the body with oxygen, while removing carbon dioxide. Some veterinarians estimate that the canine respiratory system declines in efficiency by up to 50 percent over a lifetime. Over time, the bronchial passages tend to constrict, fibrous tissue in the lungs increases, and the function of alveoli, tiny air sacs in the lungs that transmit oxygen into the bloodstream, is reduced. The airways are exposed to damage caused by inhaled allergens, foreign bodies, viruses, bacteria, and fungus, and may develop a wide range of problems.

Small- and Toy-breed dogs such as Poodles and Terriers are prone to collapsing trachea (windpipe) when this rigid structure weakens. This can happen at any age, but most often affects dogs older than six or seven. Most respiratory disorders are not age-related per se, but older dogs are often more susceptible due to decreased immune support, cancer, or other factors. For instance, an accumulation of fluid within the chest wall, called pleural effusion, interferes with the lung's ability to expand. Pleural effusion is most commonly a result of heart failure. Pneumonia, an inflammation or infection of the lungs, can also develop due to heart disease or reduced lung capacity due to age.

Immunity

The spleen, thymus, bone marrow, and lymphatic system (including lymph nodes), plus specialized cells and chemicals, make up the immune system, which protects the body against foreign invaders such as bacteria and viruses. For instance, the spleen, located in the abdomen, both filters and stores blood and immune cells while the lymphatic tissues throughout the body sift foreign material from the lymphatic fluid and blood. How well the immune system works (called immune competence) is dictated to a large degree by genetics, but it is also influenced by a lifetime of nutrition, stress, and exposure to pathogens.

The bone marrow gives birth to the various immune system cells, and the thymus gland helps these cells mature. Cell replication slows with age, and the thymus regresses as the dog matures. The immune system also produces chemicals such as interferon and interleukins, which help control immune response. "As dogs age, the immune function declines," says Dr. Carey. "Humans do this; rats and mice do this; it is part of aging." Because of lowered immune protection, aged dogs are more susceptible to disease. They get sick quicker, and have more difficulty recovering.

Dogs suffer from a number of immune-related disorders. Allergic reactions result from the overreaction of the immune system to normally "harmless" organisms or substances, such as pollen or dust. Autoimmune disease is also an immunity overreaction and misrecognition, but this time the body attacks itself rather than the outside invader. Some types of canine arthritis, called rheumatoid arthritis or autoimmune arthritis, are considered to be autoimmune diseases, but they are extremely rare.

Besides normal aging processes, the immune system can also be suppressed by disease or medical treatments for other problems. Parvovirus, endocrine abnormalities such as hypothyroidism and Cushing's disease, and medications including chemotherapeutics, radiation, and steroids used to treat cancer all can suppress the immune system.

Nerves

The brain, spinal cord, and network of nerve fibers generate and transmit electrochemical signals that connect with every inch of the body. This central nervous system (CNS) regulates and coordinates body systems, and also gives our dogs their intellect, awareness, and emotions/personality.

Age-related degeneration of the brain, deterioration of the spine that damages the spinal cord, and chemical disruptions at the cellular level that interfere with nerve conduction all play a part in nervous-system disorders affecting senior dogs. Kidney disease and liver failure, for example, may secondarily cause bizarre behavior as a result of chemical imbalances affecting the brain.

One of the most common age-related nervous system disorders is caused by degenerative disk disease that can ultimately cause partial or complete paralysis. Back problems are particularly common in long-bodied, short-legged dogs such as Dachshunds. The disks are support structures of the spine that offer flexibility and a cushion for the spinal cord. The disks are made up of tough, fibrous tissue with a jellylike center. The center tends to harden with age, and the disk loses flexibility, becoming more susceptible to damage, which, in turn, can injure the spine.

Less common, myelopathies are degenerative conditions that attack the nervous system, and affect the myelin sheath that coats nerve fibers and conducts the electrical impulses. Myelopathies are most common in aged, larger-breed dogs, and ultimately result in loss of rear-end function that affects both mobility and bladder/bowel control.

Aging Mind

As pets get older, their thought processes slow down, due in part to reduced blood flow to the brain, loss of neurons the body is unable to replace, and sometimes plaquelike deposits that interfere with function. MRI scans (magnetic resonance imaging) of the canine brain shows that it shrinks as it ages. "There's loss of neurons [nerve cells] and there's brain atrophy, and an increased amount of beta amyloid that's produced," says Dr. Hawley. Beta amyloid is a starchlike plaque typically associated with human Alzheimer's patients.

Just as with people, there are great differences in how "mentally spry" dogs remain during their golden years. While physical changes often impact

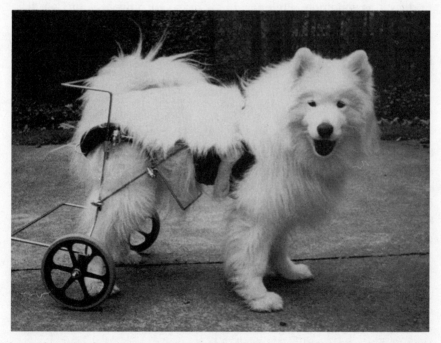

Loss of rear leg function doesn't have to slow down the dog. Wheelchairs are available for dogs of all sizes and enable them to continue to be active. *(Photo Credit: K-9 Cart Company)*

the dog's behavior—she might snap when startled because she's deaf, or she might lose housetraining due to kidney disease—the changes in an aging brain can affect both behavior and personality. A Jekyll-and-Hyde transformation can drastically impact the loving bond an owner shares with a pet. "Twenty percent of dogs go to shelters because they're 'too old' and probably because they have problems with house soiling," says Nicholas Dodman, BVMS, a professor of behavioral pharmacology at Tufts University.

Behaviorists believe many age-related behavior problems, such as separation anxiety, can be ascribed to loss of memory. "Dogs get more irritable as they forget how to respond in a dominance-subordination fashion," says Dr. Hart. Essentially, some older dogs "forget" their training and return to a puppy mind-set, to the time before they learned these lessons. Some dogs are more affected than others, and there's no way to predict how your dog will fare.

Some dogs remain incredibly sharp and connected to the world around them throughout their geriatric years. "There is a subset of older dogs that are not as successful at aging as others," says Dr. Dodman. "These dogs seem to develop something akin to Alzheimer's disease in human patients." In dogs, this condition is referred to as canine cognitive dysfunction. It is commonly characterized by memory loss that affects training, and prompts behavior problems such as separation anxiety, house soiling, and personality changes.

Reproduction

Aging dogs that have not been neutered or spayed often develop reproductive diseases. The organs that cause the most problems are the uterus and mammary glands in the female, and the prostate in the male.

Dogs do not suffer the equivalent of human menopause. Most female dogs experience estrus twice a year throughout their life, and are capable of becoming pregnant until they die. However, fertility and libido may decrease with age. For instance, rather than a typical litter of six pups they may conceive only one or two, sometimes skip a cycle, or show reduced interest in romance even during estrus.

Intact female dogs older than six are highly prone to pyometra—a life-threatening infection of the uterus. Kidney failure may be triggered by pyometra, a result of the body's efforts to fight the infection. Breast cancer is also a risk in aging unaltered female dogs.

The older they are, the greater becomes the risk for unaltered male dogs to suffer prostate problems. Infections, cysts, tumors, and enlargements that may block urine or stool are common prostate problems of aging dogs. Hind-limb lameness and/or water retention in the region can develop when the prostate enlargement blocks lymphatic drainage.

Skin and Hair

Skin is the single largest organ of the dog's body. With the fur, the outer covering provides a protective barrier from the elements, and from viruses, bacteria, and other disease-causing pathogens. The skin and fur regulate temperature, prevent dehydration, and serve as the major sensory organ for touch. The dog's skin and hair, known as the integumentary system, are also an accurate barometer of her health—what she feels on the inside is reflected on the outside.

Normal skin changes occur with age due to a lifetime of exposure to the environment and to changes in the dog's metabolism. Skin becomes thinner, less flexible, and cysts can develop from glands in the skin. The hair coat becomes duller and drier due to less oil production, and some hair, especially around the muzzle, often turns gray.

The most common skin disease among dogs is various allergies, but these are not necessarily old-age specific, although older dogs do seem to be more susceptible, particularly to fleas. Years of inflammation due to inhaled allergens, biting pests, or food ingredients may cause permanent changes in the skin. For instance, dogs with itchy skin that constantly lick themselves often develop blackened, thickened skin from saliva stains.

Calluses, particularly on the elbows and ankle region, are quite common in older large-breed dogs. They are caused by years of lying on hard or rough surfaces. Calluses can become inflamed and painful.

A number of skin and fur disorders arise as a result of other age-related disorders. Diabetes mellitus and Cushing's disease often prompt hair thinning or loss. Aging Dachshunds and Cocker Spaniels are prone to a hormonal disease called acanthosis nigricans that causes hair loss, darkened skin, and thickening of skin primarily in the armpit and chest regions.

Urinary System

Two kidneys, two ureters, a bladder, and a urethra make up the urinary system. Body wastes are filtered from the blood and removed by the kidneys. The ureters route urine from the kidneys into the bladder, which collects and stores this liquid waste until it's released from the body through the urethra as urine. Kidneys not only manage waste; they also produce a hormone called erythropoietin, which prompts the production of red blood cells and also helps regulate blood pressure.

As the dog's kidneys age the tissue deteriorates, the organs slowly shrink, and they gradually lose their ability to function efficiently. Kidney disease and failure is one of the most common diseases affecting geriatric dogs.

Other disorders of the urinary system include urinary-tract infections, and urinary stones that affect the bladder, the kidneys, or both. Infections and stones (urolithiasis) may affect dogs of any age, however, and are no more common in aging dogs than they are in youthful canines.

Aging dogs, though, can develop urinary incontinence—especially female dogs. "Urinary incontinence is problematic, especially for those animals that sleep in the bed with their people," says Bill Fortney, DVM, director of community practice at Kansas State University. This condition has no relationship to cognitive dysfunction, where the dog "forgets" training. "They just have a leaky bladder," says Dr. Fortney. The sphincter that controls the release of urine loses muscle tone, and the dog loses bladder control.

A dog's body systems do not age independently of each other. When healthy, each system provides support for every other system. When one

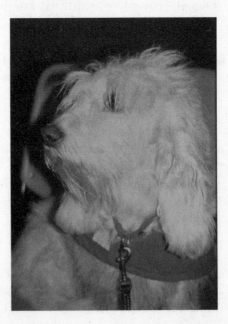

PG, a retired show dog, spends her golden years doing therapy work. *(Photo Credit: Amy D. Shojai)*

falters, it may prompt a cascade effect in multiple organs throughout the body. Whether slow or abrupt, the various changes in the different body systems collectively contribute to canine aging. By addressing a single age-related issue, you can influence and often slow the entire aging process, and help your dog age gracefully while still enjoying her golden years.

Golden Moments: Thinking Young

Nancy Lind of Chicago doesn't think of PG as being old, even though the Petit Basset Griffon Vendéen (PBGV) has celebrated her eleventh birthday. PG has received good health care, including preventive care, all her life. PG's health remains good, although she is on a special fish-and-potato diet to accommodate her food allergy. She still loves to participate just for fun, but no longer competes in agility or flyball since the racing around became too much for her.

"As they get older, they're much more prone to aches and pains," says Nancy. Her puppy, Beaner, harasses the older dog, and during roughhousing PG sometimes gets sideswiped. The PBGV breed can be predisposed to back problems because of their long, low-to-the-ground body, so PG also gets regular chiropractic adjustments.

Other accommodations Nancy has made have more to do with PG's emotional health. "She was raised in an outdoor kennel and was a show dog," says Nancy. For her first two years of life, her home was out in the middle of the country, where PG was totally surrounded by a six-foot stockade fence that kept the world at bay. "She walked nicely on a lead, she stayed in the kennel really nice, but she wasn't used to the commotion of city life," says Nancy. "That was tough on her. And as she's gotten older, she's less tolerant of stresses."

PG has always worked with children as a therapy dog with Rainbow Animal Assisted Therapy Group, and she loves it. "Once I get her in the therapy session she's great!" says Nancy. "She's relaxed, she does her work, and she enjoys the kids."

However, getting into the room can be very stressful. Several times on the way to therapy, PG became so agitated and stressed by walking down long strange hallways with doors popping open unexpectedly and all kinds of people going by that she got sick. It came to a point where PG would remember that *this* was the scary place and would be stressed before going inside. So now PG works only in settings that bypass all the upsetting hallways, doors, and people. "We go through a door right in the room with the kids and she's fine," says Nancy.

Don't dismiss a behavior change as something you must live with, suggests Nancy. "When your very active dog is no longer running around like an idiot, it's not just age. Usually they're not feeling good," says Nancy. "They don't tell you much." She believes it's vital to "listen" to what your dog tells you at any age, but especially as they get older.

CHAPTER 3

L.O.V.E. for Health

It is important to be tuned in to your pet's needs at any age, but vital when she becomes a senior citizen. You don't have to be a veterinarian to recognize when your dog is feeling under the weather. Her physical status is intimately tied with emotional and mental health, which she often expresses by way of behavior changes. These may be sudden and obvious or, more often, insidious and subtle.

A good way to remember the special needs of your older dog is to use the acronym **L.O.V.E.** That stands for *Listen with Your Heart;* *Observe for Changes;* *Visit the Veterinarian;* and *Enrich the Environment.*

LISTEN WITH YOUR HEART

Because of the love and close relationship you share, you have an advantage when it comes to knowing when something's wrong. "It's more of an intuitive thing, when they start to slow down a little bit, when they are not quite as quick on the uptake bringing you the ball, that sort of thing," says Susan G. Wynn, DVM, a holistic veterinarian in private practice in Atlanta. It's not magic—it's simply that your subconscious pays exquisite attention to the details. Never discount that odd "feeling" that something's different, not right, wrong. Simply listen with your heart—pay attention to intuition—to stay alert to what your dog needs.

Dogs can't tap us on the shoulder to get our attention. They can't say, "I hurt," or explain, "I feel thirsty all the time," or "It's hard for me to see."

"Owners always say the dog is not what she used to be, or she's sleeping all the time," says William Tranquilli, DVM. Your memory and understanding of what used to be normal when the dog was in her prime is paramount. Only by comparing today's behavior with that benchmark will you notice subtle signs that point to a decline in health. Make it a habit to observe your dog for changes, and when they occur, recognize that something may not be right.

When your intuition and observation add up to a concern, it's time to visit the veterinarian. Regular examinations are equally important, even when your dog seems to feel fine. The veterinarian can validate any concerns and help you prevent problems.

The world in which she lives shapes how your dog interacts with you. Normal aging changes can impact her physical and emotional health when she's no longer able to do the things she's grown to love. Enriching your dog's environment—that includes her nutrition, exercise, grooming, and home—will ensure she maintains a high quality of life and enjoys the time she spends with you. Feed her mind as well as her body with mental enrichment. Follow the L.O.V.E. plan to keep her healthy and happy throughout her golden years.

NORMAL VITAL SIGNS

It's important to know what the benchmark "normal" readings are for your dog so that you are alerted to a change that might point to a health problem.

- Temperature: ranges between 99.5 degrees to 102.5 degrees.
- Hydration: Scruff test—loose skin on the neck should immediately spring back when grasped and released, and a delay indicates dehydration.
- Blood Circulation/Pressure: Capillary refill time of 1 to 2 seconds is normal. Firmly press the flat of a finger against the dog's gum, then release, and time how long it takes the pink color to return to the whitened finger-shaped mark. A delay indicates dehydration, low blood pressure, or even shock.
- Heart Rate: Small dogs, 70 to 180 beats per minute; dogs over 20 pounds, 60 to 140 beats per minute.
- Respiration: 10 to 30 breaths per minute.

OBSERVE FOR CHANGES: HOME HEALTH ALERTS

It bears repeating: You know your dog best. Therefore, in almost all cases, you will be the first to notice when something is wrong. That's because healthy aging dogs see the veterinarian only a couple of times a year, while you live with her every day.

Close proximity to your pet allows you to immediately notice any changes that can point to a potential health problem. The major disadvantage of this closeness is that you may overlook subtle changes, or those that have a slow, gradual onset. Veterinarians call sudden problems "acute," and those are the easiest for owners to spot.

Conditions that develop slowly over a long period of time, called chronic problems, are more insidious. Changes of a chronic nature creep up on you, day by day, in such small increments that you aren't likely to notice anything's wrong. By the time a problem becomes obvious, the disease may have been simmering for months or even years, and the damage may be permanent.

One of the best ways to stay on top of things is to create a log of your dog's normal behaviors. Like the health screening tests performed by the veterinarian, a home health report card provides you with a baseline measure against which to compare even subtle changes in your dog's health. And in the future, should your dog be diagnosed with a particular condition, a home health report card can also help you measure how the treatment works. That in turn helps the veterinarian make informed decisions if adjustments to the therapy are needed.

Once you have your list, and a benchmark description of "normal," use the home health report card to review and check for any changes on a monthly basis. If your dog has been diagnosed with a disease for which she's receiving treatment, a weekly or even daily check to monitor changes may be better.

Behavior Cues

Generate a list of as many of your dog's normal behaviors as possible. The categories will vary somewhat from dog to dog. Be specific. Examples of categories follow, but don't limit yourself to my suggestions. If your dog swims every day, for example, or enjoys chasing bunnies, include that as a category and describe her routine. Any changes to routine might indicate a health concern that needs attention. For instance, if she digs in her sandbox every single day at three o'clock when the kids get home from school, and suddenly loses all interest in the game, perhaps her joints hurt too much from arthritis to play.

Favorite Activity: Describe how she plays—for example, if she loves Frisbee, does she fetch? Make mad, leaping catches? Play keep-away? Bring you the toy to incite a game? How often does she ask to play? How long does the game typically last? How does she move—at a run, trot, or walk? Bounding like a rubber ball, or sedately strolling? Does she like to dig, or to chew on chew toys? *Activity monitoring can alert you to painful arthritic changes.*

Vocabulary: All dogs learn certain words—what are your dog's favorites (*outside, food, walk* . . .), and how does she react to hearing them? *A change in reaction to favorite words may indicate hearing loss, or cognitive dysfunction.*

Vocalizations: Describe what circumstances prompt barks or other vocalizations. Perhaps she goes nuts when the doorbell rings, or the neighbor cat visits. How long do vocalizations last? What do they sound like? Howls, yaps, whines, growls? *Cognitive/memory changes, hearing loss, and dimming eyesight can change how the dog vocalizes.*

Interactions/Personality: How does she get along with the other pets in the household? (describe her relationship to each one.) Detail her typical reaction to strangers—never met one? Growls and suspicion? *Personality changes may indicate sensory loss—she's startled more easily when deaf or blind and reacts accordingly. She may also become short-tempered from chronic pain.*

Sleep Cycles: When does she sleep, and for how long? Does she have a favorite spot? Sofa, the floor, your bed? What's her temperature preference— cool threshold of the front door, or puddle of sunshine? *Painful joints may prevent her from reaching favorite resting spots on the bed, and prompt her to seek out sunny spots and sleep for longer periods. Metabolic changes can influence temperature perception and sleep rates. Cognitive dysfunction often reverses sleep cycles so she's awake at night and sleeps during the day.*

Habits/Routines: What is her day like? Does she wake the kids at the same time each day? Meet you at the front door after work? Beg for a nightly twenty-minute walk? Is she the leader of the pack on the agility course? *Loss of hearing or eyesight, painful joints, brain changes, and organ dysfunction may all change routines.*

Body Warnings

Generate a list of as many of your dog's normal body functions as possible. Be as specific as possible. Examples of categories follow, but don't limit yourself to my suggestions.

Appetite: Does she have a favorite food? Is she finicky or a glutton? How much does she eat (measure the amount), and at what time of the day? *Missing one meal usually won't hurt her, but an aging dog shouldn't go longer than twenty-four hours without eating. A change in appetite points to a variety of problems, from metabolic change to chronic pain or organ dysfunction.*

Weight Loss/Gain: How much does she weigh? Is she normal, under-, or overweight? *Fluctuations in weight can be a sign of pain, diabetes mellitus, Cushing's disease, problems of the liver, kidneys, or heart, or dental disease.*

Water Intake: How often does the water bowl empty? Measure how much water goes in the bowl and the amount left at the end of the day to see how much on average she drinks in a day. *Increased thirst is a classic sign of diabetes and kidney failure as well as other organ problems.*

Urination: What color is the urine? Count the number of times she urinates in a day. How often does she have "accidents"? *Lighter than normal could mean her kidneys aren't concentrating efficiently, while darker than normal may indicate dehydration. Increased urination often results from increased water intake, and may also prompt more housebreaking lapses. Accidents could also be a sign of urinary incontinence. "Forgetting" to ask to go outside may indicate memory problems. Inability to properly "pose" and squat or leg-cock may be due to joint pain, and prompt the dog to delay bathroom breaks.*

Defecation: What is the color/consistency of the feces? Count how many bowel movements she produces each day. Does she ever have "accidents"? *Changes in the frequency of elimination and/or consistency of the stool point to potential digestive system problems. It may also indicate memory loss—she can't remember to ask to go out—or problems with mobility—it hurts to move/pose so he delays elimination.*

Skin and Fur: What color is her skin? Is it free of dandruff, sores, and lumps or bumps? Is the fur full, thick, and lustrous? *Metabolic changes are often reflected in the appearance of the skin and hair coat. Any lump or bump in an old dog is a potential risk for cancer.*

Eyes: Are her eyes clear, with no discharge or watering? *Squinting or pawing at watery eyes indicates pain, and changes in the appearance of the eye may point to eye diseases such as cataracts or glaucoma.*

Ears: Do her ears smell fresh? Are they clean? Does she scratch them or shake her head? *Stinky, dirty, or itchy ears point to an infection.*

Nose: What color is the nose leather? Is it moist and smooth, or dry and chapped? Is there any discharge? *Nasal discharge can be a sign of systemic infection. Changes to the nose leather, as in the skin, can indicate metabolic changes or even nasal dermoid cancer.*

Respiration: Is her breathing regular and easy, or does she gasp and strain to get air? Does she have bad breath? *Exercise intolerance, characterized by panting/gasping and refusing further activity, is a sign of heart disease. Dogs often sit with a characteristic elbows-out posture to relieve the pressure on their chest when they breathe. Bad breath may indicate periodontal disease, diabetes, or kidney disease.*

Gait/Movement: Does she arise easily from sitting or lying down? Does she hold up or favor a leg? Refuse to climb stairs, jump onto or off of favorite furniture, or fear the dark? Does she have trouble navigating unknown territory? *Gait or activity changes are strong indications of painful arthritis. They may also indicate vision loss.*

VISIT THE VETERINARIAN: WELL-PET EXAMS

An annual checkup for your dog is a good idea whatever her age. In the past, annual vaccinations were recommended, and that was a good reminder to get a physical examination at the same time. More recent studies indicate that annual vaccines may not be necessary. However, since dogs age so much more quickly than people do, an annual physical—or "well-pet" exam—is essential to ensure that she maintains good health.

The well-pet exam becomes even more important for aging dogs, because they have fewer reserves and can become ill literately overnight. Each year, mature dogs age the equivalent of about seven human years, so waiting twelve months between checkups leaves them at risk for major health changes. A twice-yearly visit for dogs over the age of eight makes more sense. That's the equivalent to a middle-aged person getting a physical about every three years, says Dr. Tranquilli, which is still pushing it a bit. "It makes all the sense in the world to get more aggressive with checkups, and for the veterinarian to ask appropriate questions with regard to overall behavior changes," he says.

A veterinarian has a more difficult time diagnosing problems if he sees the pet only when she's sick and has no way to compare to well-pet behavior, especially when looking for subtle disease. "I want to see the pet every year so I've seen him when he's healthy," says Steven L. Marks, DVM. "If something changes, I want to pick it up early."

A complete physical should include an oral exam, says Bill Gengler, DVM. "You may not be able to do an in-depth exam until the animal's asleep, but at least you can advise the owner that yes, there's halitosis; yes, there's gingivitis; and there's calculus [tartar] on the teeth, so we need to get it off."

The veterinarian will listen to the dog's heart and lungs, check her eyes, ears, and teeth, examine her for parasites, and make a note of any behavior changes you might have noticed that could indicate a problem.

"As these animals get older, one starts looking at their liver, their intestinal tract, their kidneys, at their heart and various body systems, looking for those organs that could be failing," says Johnny D. Hoskins, DVM, an internist and specialist in aging pets. "The number one cause of death in older dogs is cancer." Looking at the outside of the dog and listening to her breathing and heart won't detect organ failures or cancer. Geriatric screening tests help veterinarians go beyond the hands-on exam and take a look at the dog from the inside out.

Screening Tests

Evaluating the blood and urine may uncover abnormalities that otherwise would not be found until it is too late for treatment to help. Something as simple as a urinalysis, that examines the content and volume of the urine, can alert you to canine kidney disease, liver disease, Cushing's disease, diabetes mellitus, and other health problems.

The best time to have the first screening tests is when your dog is between seven and ten years of age and in good health, to establish a "normal" baseline against which future tests can be compared. "If we can catch these things much earlier in the course of disease, we can do a lot better job by controlling it or getting rid of it," says Rhonda L. Schulman, DVM, an internist at the University of Illinois. In addition to routine blood and urine screening, some veterinarians also recommend chest and abdominal X rays or ultrasound to make sure the organs are normal.

Every dog is an individual, and there are slight variations between dogs as to what constitutes normal. "What we consider a normal range of values is normal for about 95 percent of people," says Dr. Marks. "So 5 percent of normal animals and people will be outside that range." Therefore, having a baseline test is particularly helpful to determine your dog's normal range, as a comparison for the future.

The veterinarian can get an idea of the health of a variety of organs by looking at specific factors in the blood. A complete blood count (CBC) measures the components that make up the blood. For instance, the hematocrit (HCT), or packed cell volume, is the ratio of red cells to total blood volume. A lower-than-normal HCT indicates anemia, while an elevated HCT is an indication of dehydration or of chronic obstructive pulmonary disease. The CBC also typically measures the percentages of the various white blood cells. High or low numbers can indicate anything from infections or tissue damage to cancer or autoimmune disorders.

A biochemical profile measures the various chemicals, vitamins, minerals, enzymes, and other compounds in the bloodstream. Blood urea nitrogen (BUN) is the by-product of protein metabolism, and the BUN level is a good measure of kidney health. The liver does so many things that many diseases affect it. Therefore, the liver is a wonderful health barometer for the rest of the body. For instance, bile acids produced in the liver act to absorb fat, so abnormal blood levels of bile acids indicate liver problems. Enzymes produced by the liver are very sensitive, and the levels in the

BLOOD VALUES

Blood Count	Normal Range
Red Blood Cell Count (RBC)	4.8 to 9.3 million/microliter
Hemoglobin (Hgb)	12.1 to 20.3 grams/deciliter
Hematocrit (HCT)	37 to 55 percent
Mean Corpuscular Volume (MCV)	58 to 79 femtoliter
Mean Corpuscular Hemoglobin (MCH)	19 to 28 picograms
Mean Corpuscular Hemoglobin Concentration (MCHC)	30 to 38 grams/deciliter
White Blood Cell Count (WBC)	4.0 to 15.5 thousand/ microliter
Neutrophils	60 to 77 percent
Lymphocytes	12 to 30 percent
Monocytes	3 to 10 percent
Eosinophils	2 to 10 percent
Platelets	170 to 400 thousand/ microliter

bloodstream will go up if the liver is damaged, says Cynthia R. Leveille-Webster, DVM, an internist at Tufts University. But elevations can also indicate other diseases. "Probably 80 percent of the time you'll find another disease causing that enzyme to go up," she says. "It might indicate Cushing's disease, because that's a very common old-dog disease."

It's important to remember, though, that many of these tests are simply for screening the *possibility* of a problem. If a liver enzyme is elevated, more specific diagnostic evaluations, such as X rays and ultrasound, are required to figure out the exact cause, says Dr. Marks.

Checking biochemical abnormalities alone ignores the total animal. When your dog feels great, but has an abnormal lab value on the blood work, Dr. Marks says you have a choice. You can aggressively pursue the cause with further diagnostics, or you can wait a month to repeat the test and, if the result is still abnormal, then go further. "I'm not really a fan of saying we have to do *all* these tests on *all* pets over eight years old," he says. It depends on the owner, the comfort level of the veterinarian, and most especially on the health status of your individual dog. Still, early detection offers the best hope of controlling any illness.

ENRICH THE ENVIRONMENT

Dogs older than seven often have the constitution and attitude of much younger animals. Your dog doesn't know she should feel or act any differently the day she turns seven. Expect the best of her, give her the best help possible, and there's no reason why she shouldn't enjoy a rewarding and vital life well into her golden years.

Health maintenance is paramount for seniors, and mirrors that of youngsters. The help you give her includes good nutrition, exercise, grooming, environmental accommodations, and mental stimulation.

Nutrition

How do you choose the best diet for your aging dog? "There isn't any one best food," says Sarah K. Abood, DVM, a clinical nutritionist at Michigan State University. A number of therapeutic diets address specific diseases, such as kidney failure, once the dog has been diagnosed. Dr. Abood says that the therapeutic diets for a given condition are pretty similar no matter who makes them. "When animals do better on one over the other, that's an individual animal variation; that's not a diet difference," she says. "If the dog refuses to eat the diet, it doesn't matter what magical foo-foo you have in there, or how modified it is. If they don't recognize it as food, it's not going to do the job you want it to do."

Check with your veterinarian for the best time to change your dog to a "senior" diet. Some very well conditioned older dogs that still bounce around like puppies may not need to switch to a "senior" diet as early as the seven-year average, says Dr. Abood. There are exceptions, but Dan Carey, DVM, of the Iams Company says the body requirements of an aging dog usually change before there are visible signs of aging. Your veterinarian can best judge the timing after reviewing routine blood and urine screening tests. The newest senior-label diets are designed to support the dog during these changes so she maintains that puppylike behavior.

You have basically two choices when it comes to feeding your dog, says Gary Landsberg, DVM, a behaviorist at Doncaster Animal Clinic in Thornhill, Ontario—do-it-yourself diets or commercial products. "People aren't entirely wrong when they talk about feeding *all-natural* or even raw-food diets, and talk about adding vitamins and natural supplements to the diet," he says. A relatively new pet food company, Steve's Real Food (www.stevesrealfood.com), has created commercially prepared raw-food diets that are frozen or freeze-dried, in an attempt to provide a safe and nutritious natural alternative. "The idea of getting ingredients that act as natural antioxidants is a good idea," says Dr. Lansberg, "but I don't think there's any evidence that raw meats are any better than cooked meats."

Today, commercial pet food companies recognize the benefits of natural ingredients. "For now, the premium dog food companies are the ones who hire the nutritionists," says Dr. Landsberg. "They are the ones who are doing the research to enhance their food and make it better, so I stick to the premium dog foods."

Homemade diets fall under the "therapeutic diet" category. If you plan to feed them, they should be designed by a veterinary nutritionist to ensure they're right for your individual dog, says Dr. Wynn.

Because a senior dog typically burns less energy, lower calories are at the heart of most senior diets. "A lot of them also have added antioxidants, or added protein, or added this or that," says Dr. LaFlamme. It's essential that the diet meet the needs of the individual pet. You don't want to be feeding your dog the equivalent of rocket fuel when she's a couch potato. Conversely, if your fourteen-year-old dog is still a dynamo, she'll need more calories to keep her healthy.

Senior diets typically are designed to be highly digestible to compensate for those animals whose digestive systems may no longer be as efficient, says Blake Hawley, DVM. "By manipulating the nutrients, we have the ability to allow them to better absorb things." Other considerations may be added fiber to keep bowels healthy, or softer textures for dogs suffering from dental disease.

Ask your veterinarian to recommend a diet. If you choose a commercial senior diet, the label should say the food is "complete and balanced" in accordance with guidelines established by AAFCO (Association of Animal Feed Control Officials).

Don't neglect water. As they age, dogs tend to stop drinking as much water, which makes them more prone to dehydration. It may be harder for her to make the trip clear across the house for a drink, so add a couple of water bowls in different places to make it more convenient.

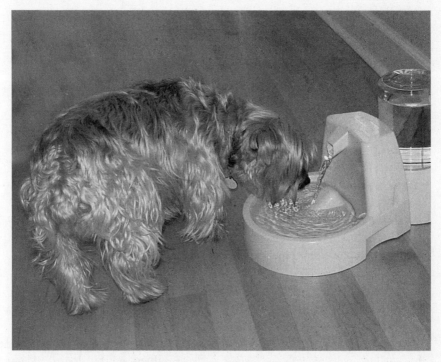

The most important nutrient of all is water. Dehydration can be a problem with aging dogs. Providing fresh water at all times, in a convenient dispenser, encourages dogs to drink. The Drinkwell Pet Fountain is available at www.vetventures.com. *(Photo Credit: © Veterinary Ventures)*

FEEDING FOR HEALTH

It is impossible to list all of the various dog foods available for mature dogs, but you can start with the following list to see if one or more fits your dog's needs:

- Eukanuba Senior
- Hill's Science Diet Canine Senior
- IVD Select Care Canine Mature Formula
- Nutro Max Senior
- Nutro Natural Choice Senior
- Precise Senior Formula
- Purina Dog Chow Senior 7+
- Wysong Senior

Exercise

Exercise is vital to dogs of all ages, but particularly as they get older. When your pet is a youngster, twenty minutes aerobic exercise twice a day helps keep her physically fit as well as mentally alert—and out of trouble. Behavior problems often develop when a dog doesn't have enough to do to work off her energy.

When your pet is a senior citizen, it takes an extra effort to get her moving at the same level. Remember to include warm-up exercises and cool-down stretches to prevent pulled muscles. Invite your dog into a "play bow" with head down and tail up, for a natural stretch. After exercise, give her a gentle massage to help her cool down.

Simple movement gives her a much-needed healthy edge. Muscles that aren't used atrophy. Muscle mass is the buffer the dog needs to maintain health and recover from injury or disease, and so muscle loss can have risky consequences.

The joints help feed themselves by spreading nutrients with the pumping action of their movement. A reduction in movement allows the joints to get rusty and become less efficient, and can speed the progression of arthritis. Painful arthritis, in turn, makes the dog reluctant to move—and the vicious cycle of reduced exercise also predisposes the dog to weight gain. Obesity puts more strain on the already painful joints, making the dog even more reluctant to move her furry tail. Obesity also predisposes dogs to metabolic disorders such as diabetes mellitus.

As she ages, your dog may not be physically capable of maintaining the same level of exercise she enjoyed as a youthful athlete. Painful joints aren't helped by the concussive action of leaps and jumps, so you may need to carefully control her exercise.

Rather than a jog on hard surfaces, take her for a controlled walk on the leash around the block, or up the hill. Use food or toy rewards to tempt her interest. Terriers especially enjoy games that involve chasing, and a favorite stuffed animal dragged along the grass in the backyard may spark interest. For small dogs, walking once or twice around the family room or up and down the stairs may be more than adequate. Many dogs love going for a ride, so use this reward as a bribe to entice her to walk down the driveway to reach the car.

Dogs obsessed with toys such as the Frisbee or tennis ball often are fetching fools, and easy to entice into exercise. They don't always know when to quit, though, and can easily hurt themselves if they overdo. Instead of tossing the toy high in the air, keep the Frisbee or ball low to the ground. That gives them the thrill of the chase and the fun of the game without prompting dangerous leaps that could hurt them. Make sure she has adequate time to catch her breath between mad dashes. Smaller dogs may relish a game of fetch inside the house, with a soft-sided toy.

Another good game for exercise is a modified "keep-away" that keeps the dog moving back and forth between two or more people. Be sure you allow her to "catch" the toy after every few tosses, so she doesn't lose interest in the game. You can play keep-away using foam Frisbees or soft stuffed animals inside the house with a small dog.

Swimming is an ideal low-impact aerobic exercise for many dogs that enjoy the water, says Dr. Wynn. "But when they're fourteen years old isn't the time to teach them to swim," she cautions. Retriever breeds such as Labradors are natural water athletes who enjoy fetching toys from the pool, or paddling in shallow water alongside the beach. Small dogs such as miniature Dachshunds may benefit from regular swimming in the bathtub.

The best idea is to maintain a level of aerobic exercise the dog enjoys, so you don't have to fight her every step of the way. Establish a daily routine for your dog—ten to twenty minutes every morning and evening is a good target.

Don't wait for her to ask you to go for a walk. At the scheduled time, take the leash to her, wake her from a nap if necessary, and get her up and moving. Dogs will certainly sleep all day if given nothing more interesting to do! The great advantage of a regular exercise program is that your dog will feel better, act younger, and remain healthier for much longer. When this is something you can do together, it also enhances the bond you share.

Physical Therapy

"Physical therapy especially for geriatrics is absolutely essential," says Signe Beebe, DVM. This is true whether your dog suffers from an illness and needs help recovering, or is completely well and you want to help her maintain that healthy edge. Most physical therapy methods are easy to do at home and involve no cost. For example, standing exercises, slow walks, swim therapy, stair climbing, treadmill activity, wheelbarrowing (forelimb activity), dancing (rear-limb activity), jogging, sit-to-stand exercises, pulling/carrying weights, ball playing, and sling walking are commonly used therapeutic exercises, says Paul M. Shealy, DVM, a veterinary surgeon and small-animal rehab specialist in South Carolina and Georgia.

Professional massage and physical therapists available at some veterinary practices can offer more involved treatment when necessary. "Progressive veterinary specialists now consider it antiquated to perform surgery only to place patients in confinement for weeks or months for the healing process to ensue," says Dr. Shealy. Many conditions can avoid surgery simply by using physical therapy, and nonsurgical conditions benefit as well, says Dr. Shealy.

Physical therapy can include cold packs to decrease pain and swelling, and heat therapy, which increases circulation and healing, relaxes skeletal muscles, reduces muscle spasm, and decreases pain and joint stiffness. Exercise helps improve balance, coordination, endurance, and flexibility. Massage increases blood flow and removes lymphatic drainage from injured tissues. Supportive devices range from braces that help protect a nerve-damaged leg, to wheeled carts that cradle the rear end of a paralyzed dog and allow her to get around.

Dogs that are already overweight, suffering from arthritis, or recovering from surgery also benefit from exercise in the form of rehabilitation or physical therapy. Your veterinarian may suggest a program to help the dog slim down, regain mobility, and reduce pain. The mental stimulation will also improve her quality of life. Muscle that's lost through disuse will never be regained, so don't delay getting your dog back on her feet and back into life.

Start slowly, and gradually build up the duration of exercise. An obese dog may do well to walk down the sidewalk to the mailbox and back within thirty minutes. If she stops and refuses to go on, listen to her. Give her the break, let her rest, and then urge her to continue.

What if your dog is blind, or has some other condition that makes her reluctant to move? "Sometimes we'll do passive range of motion," says

James L. Cook, DVM. That at least keeps the muscles and joints flexible. "You can kind of wheelbarrow them, or do dancing with them, so you work the front legs and then the hind legs," he suggests. Take care not to overdo, and avoid manipulating or flexing the dog's joints yourself—let it be under her power, so you don't overextend and injure her. Some blind dogs will follow their noses for a smelly treat. Get creative in tempting her to move.

"I think massage is so critical; they really feel better when you work them," says Dr. Susan G. Wynn. Massage can be an acquired taste, though, and it will likely take repeated sessions before your dog decides massage at your hands is the best thing in the world. Many large veterinary practices now have a massage therapist or physical therapy specialist available to work with clients and their animals. "Basically you're looking for sore spots, and you work at the level of pressure that the animal can tolerate, so you don't cause pain," says Dr. Wynn.

Massage targets the muscles and tendons. Injury to these tissues causes a release of chemicals that prompt inflammation, pain, spasms, abnormal contractions, and tightness of the muscles and tendons. That makes it even more painful to move. Massage applies varying pressure to these areas to increase blood circulation. That helps nourish the tissue, relieve pain, and promote healing, and is particularly helpful for dogs recovering from illness, injury, or surgery.

Different techniques work best for different purposes, and some require special training so you don't accidentally injure your dog. Keep massage sessions to ten or fifteen minutes long. Once a day is plenty, says Dr. Wynn. Let your dog tell you when she's had enough. Firm, even-pressured palm strokes are called effleurage. This technique helps the dog relax when you stroke slowly from the head to the tail, and down the legs to the feet. Use effleurage to begin and progress to fingertip massage. Use the flat of your extended fingers held close together, and rub in a circular pattern with enough pressure to move muscle beneath the skin. Petrissage uses a deeper technique that kneads the muscle to relax the tissue, promote blood flow, and stimulate the lymph system and a release of toxins. The dog must be fully relaxed for this massage technique to be beneficial. Fingers grasp and gently squeeze, roll, and compress the muscle beside the bone, in a bread-kneading motion. Finish each session with the effleurage technique—a head-to-tail petting session that leaves her feeling good.

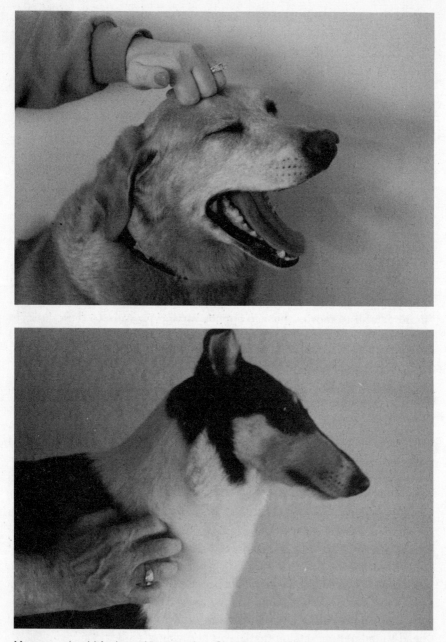

Massage should feel good to your dog. Start out with flat-hand strokes, proceed to fingertip strokes, and for deeper massage, you can use your knuckles. Remember to avoid massaging directly on top of bones—that hurts! Massage the muscles on either side of bones.   *(Photo Credit: "Dog Massage" by Maryjean Ballner)*

Golden Moments: A Decade of Flying High!

Gail Mirabella wanted to find an all-around doggy companion to keep her company on hikes, mountain biking, and rock climbing trips. When she saw an ad in the paper for farm dogs, she used her whole tax return to buy a pup for $200.

Austin, an Australian Shepherd, became her constant companion. Gail didn't have a car, so she strapped on Rollerblades, taught the dog to wear a harness, and Austin towed her all around Boulder. "He came to work with me at a mall pet store, we went bungee jumping together, and he's ridden in hot-air balloons—we're inseparable," says Gail.

They moved to Connecticut in 1996, and their life changed forever when a stranger happened to see Gail and Austin playing with a Frisbee. "She said we should compete. I didn't know about Frisbee competition," says Gail.

At their first event, the judge was so impressed with Austin that he wanted to buy him. "I said no!" says Gail. "So he asked if he could coach me." Gail had no doubts about her dog's abilities, but says she had to learn how to throw better.

Practice paid off. "In 1997 I was the first woman to win the Northeast

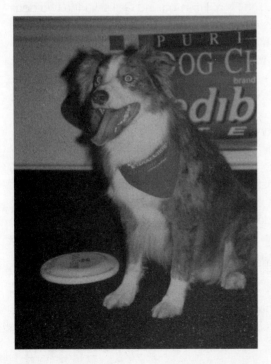

Austin has always been an athlete. Regular exercise, along with good health care, keeps him acting and feeling years younger than his actual age of ten. *(Photo Credit: Amy D. Shojai)*

Regional, and went to my first world final," she says. Her coach and mentor, Ed Jacabowski, cried, he was so happy. In less than a year, Austin's phenomenal natural talent brought him to a level most dogs never achieve.

Since then, "Air Austin" has become a celebrity and canine model featured in photo shoots, has competed in a total of three world finals, and at ten years old has retired from competition. Today, Austin and Gail tour the country with the Purina Incredible Dogs program and give Frisbee demonstrations. "We do about ten events a year. Each event is up to four days long with three shows a day," says Gail. "He always gives 110 percent, no matter what. He'll grab a Frisbee, carry it around, and say 'Throw it, throw it!' and heat up the crowd," says Gail.

Gail expects Austin should be able to continue performing demos for at least a couple more years, although she limits his vaulting and extreme jumps to prevent potential injuries. She notices that Austin's speed is still there, but he doesn't jump as high as he used to. "I can see the frustration on his face when he tries," she says. "We still compete in flyball, and Austin is the oldest dog on the team—and he's still one of the fastest."

Part of his good health comes from Austin's competitive nature. Gail has five dogs, and these days Austin is the senior dog in charge. As enforcer he keeps even the rowdy youngsters in line. He also performs in tandem with his two-and-a-half-year-old son, High Flyin' Houston and Gail says the two dogs push each other to excel. When Houston turned in a faster flyball finish than his dad, Gail said Austin eventually figured out a way to get faster. He perfected a "box turn" technique to shave off time in the race.

The two dogs often work as a team for the Frisbee demonstrations. "They're so happy to be together. Daddy grooms his son every night, cleans his ears and eyes; it's very cute," says Gail. "Having a younger dog in an older dog's life helps keep them young."

Besides a youthful sidekick, what are the keys to Austin's mature vitality? Diet is very important because he burns so much energy. "He also goes to a chiropractor and acupuncturist once a month for maintenance," says Gail. That takes care of any bruises or strains from work or play, such as swimming in the lake or racing up and down trails. The exercise keeps Austin in tiptop form. "I had to ask the vet once about some lumps, and found out they're his abdominal muscles. Austin's got a six-pack!"

Gail says you shouldn't think of your dog as being old, or treat him any differently. Take him for that walk; keep the weight off; don't slow down just because he's had another birthday. "People make excuses—'He's old now and doesn't need that much exercise,' " she says, "But that's kind of like putting the dog in a nursing home and giving up on him. You've just got to keep them young at heart and mind."

Her dogs come first in Gail's life. "I love Austin. Besides my father, he's the longest relationship I've ever had with a guy," she says. The ten-year-old Aussie continues to wow the crowds with his high-flying leaps and joyful athletics, but Gail remains his biggest fan. "Boyfriends will come and go, but my dog is always going to be there."

Grooming

Good grooming benefits the aging dog's physical and emotional health. The skin is the outer reflection of inner health. Keeping the fur clean, combed, and tangle-free prevents fleas, ticks, and fungus infections such as ringworm from causing problems. Grooming is also a great opportunity to give your dog an all-over check for any stray lumps, bumps, or sores that hide beneath the fur coat. Early detection offers the best chance for diagnosing and effectively treating tumors, for example.

Good grooming includes taking care of the eyes, ears, and teeth. "Just keeping their eyes clean, particularly in the longhaired breeds of dogs, is important," says Harriet Davidson, DVM. "It's not true that hair grows over the animal's eyes to protect them. We don't want hairs rubbing on the cornea, causing irritation." Keep hair trimmed away or pulled back.

Excessive tearing needs to be evaluated by the veterinarian, says Dr. Davidson, unless you know your dog is a breed (Pekingese, for example) known to have watery eyes. "Tears are salty and they will cause irritation on the skin," she says. Use a clean cloth and warm water on the skin and eyewash such as sterile saline solution to rinse out the eye.

Make a point of looking inside your dog's ears at least once a week. Dogs with stand-up "prick" ears tend to have fewer problems because the air is able to circulate and keep the ears dry. Drop-eared dogs, especially those with very furry ears (Cocker Spaniels, for example) are much more prone to infections because bacteria like moist, warm places to grow. Keep the fur trimmed around the ears.

Brushing your dog's teeth every day—or as often as you can—is the best way to prevent oral disease, says Dr. Gengler. Home-care chlorhexidine-based products are particularly helpful. "Chlorhexidine is an excellent product to prevent and treat periodontal disease because it kills the bacteria [that causes plaque]," he says. "It's used as an oral rinse, and it's combined into toothpaste."

AGE-DEFYING TIPS

Dogs with long floppy ears are much more prone to chronic ear infection.
Once a week, try taping the ears "open" so they can air out more easily,
to prevent problems from developing.

- Fold the floppy ears over the top of the dog's head, and tape them
  with nonstick bandage tape that won't pull his fur.
- Distract your dog with a toy for at least half an hour—two hours'
  airing out is even better.

Dr. Gengler believes it's as important to teach young animals about dental care at home as it is to teach them about a leash. "You can make amazing strides toward health and a long, quality life span by brushing their teeth," he says. Not everyone can manage that, of course, and chew toys designed for canine dental health may be an alternative. Take care in your choices, though. Dr. Gengler says the hard nylon-type bones, cow hooves, ice cubes, and real bones are the top four causes of dogs breaking teeth. For dental health, stick to rawhide chews, rubber-type "dental" chew toys, or rope-type products, and supervise the dog's recreational chewing.

Accommodations

As dogs age, you may need to make adjustments to their environment to protect them and to maintain their emotional health. Environmental accommodations will vary from pet to pet. The important point is to make changes that help your dog continue to function in as normal a fashion as possible.

For example, blind dogs will be unable to see changes to their surroundings. They memorize the house and navigate by means of a mental map. Rearranging the furniture may leave them lost in their own home. It may also leave them open to the danger of falling down stairs, becoming trapped in out-of-the-way rooms, burned in the fireplace, or drowned in the hot tub. Baby gates work extremely well to create movable barriers to protect blind or unsteady dogs from falling down stairs, for instance.

People feel a lot of empathy and distress for their pet's loss of hearing or sight, says George M. Strain, DVM. "Don't worry that the dog is suffering; there's nothing to suggest that they are," he says. "You just have to protect them from dangers they no longer detect." It's very important that you maintain the status quo for dogs with sensory impairments, and provide barriers to keep them away from the dangers they can no longer see and avoid.

Similarly, arthritic pets often need help to continue their normal routine, because they aren't as flexible or able to manage leaps. Very large dogs
may have trouble getting up after a nap, and a makeshift tummy sling gives
them the boost up that they need. The carriers made to transport firewood
have handles on each end and are ideal for big dogs, says Lynne Rutenberg,
a professional breeder of Newfoundlands. A long towel may also work.

Baby gates or playpens can humanely confine dogs when necessary,
while allowing them to still see and feel connected to the people in the next
room. For example, older dogs who become incontinent won't be welcome
on the carpet—but lining a playpen with disposable diapers, or providing a
small bathroom with an "emergency" area makes accidents less stressful to
the dogs and the owners.

Those pets used to sleeping on your bed become distressed when
they're no longer able to manage the leap. Getting in and out of the car can
become a major issue, especially for large dogs.

A wide range of products is now available to make pets more comfortable and maintain their quality of life. For example, there are ramps for
getting into and out of cars; stair steps for easy sofa access; elevated feeding
stations to accommodate an animal with a stiff neck who can't bend down;
even mattresses with warming elements to keep old bones and stiff joints
limber. Pet doors can be added so her more frequent potty breaks are readily accommodated whether you're home or not.

But you don't have to spend money to make positive changes in the environment that help your dog, and you. Move the footstool closer to the

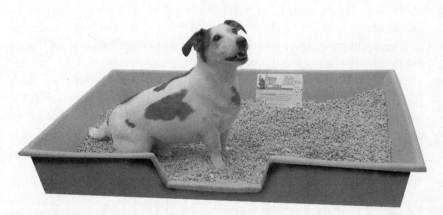

Dogs can be trained to use indoor bathroom facilities, and this can come in handy
with aging or incontinent pets. Canine litter products are available, such as Puppy
Go Potty.   (Photo Credit: © Absorption Corp and Puppy Go Potty)

sofa so she has an extra step to get up and down. Situate a study lamp over the dog's bed for a warmer resting place. Set the dog's food bowls on a box so she can reach more easily. Cover sofa cushions (or the doggy bed) first with a plastic garbage bag, then put the fabric cover back on, so any "accident" won't go into the cushion itself, but can be more easily cleaned just by removing and washing the cover.

You can even make your own inexpensive booster steps. "Cut sheets of Styrofoam insulation to the proper lengths, and use Liquid Nails to glue them together," suggests Rutenberg. Home-improvement stores stock these sheets, which can be cut and stacked to form shallow steps in whatever dimensions you need—to help your dog reach the sofa or bed, look out the window, get in the car, or onto the porch. Once the steps are glued together, you can cover them with a washable sheet and use string or rubber bands to hold the sheet tight against each step. The Styrofoam steps are lightweight, mobile, and easily cleaned.

Exercising the Mind

One of the most important contributions you can make to your aging dog's quality of life is helping to keep her mind active. The old saying, "Use it or lose it!" applies for both physical and mental activity. The canine mind that is not challenged on a regular basis becomes stagnant, bored, and less engaged in the world around it—including you!

Include brain-teasing games in your daily routine to keep her mind agile. Ask her to bring you her ball, for example, or play hide-and-seek with treats that she sees you stash beneath the pillow. She doesn't have to be able to see or hear to play these games—put her nose to use with a particularly pungent treat. Liver and fishy treats work particularly well, or if she's toy-oriented, a favorite ball may work.

First show her the treat, and let her have one. Next, allow her to watch you "hide" the treat in an obvious location—maybe in your shoe, or on the bottom shelf of the bookcase. Get her excited by encouraging her with a command such as, "Find it! Find it!" and then praise her extravagantly when she does. Once she learns the rules of the game—that she's supposed to find hidden treats—you can increase the degree of difficulty.

Puzzle toys are available that dispense food as the dog manipulates them, and can keep your dog engaged and thinking. These work best with dogs that are food-motivated. Some have bells incorporated in them, and will be particularly attractive to blind dogs.

Terriers especially enjoy games of chase and capture, and you can use a stuffed toy tied onto a ribbon to entice her to "hunt." Try dragging the toy underneath a sheet, blanket, or throw pillow for her to burrow after and capture.

Have her practice obedience lessons, never mind that she's no longer competing—or that she never entered a show. You can certainly teach old dogs new tricks, particularly something they already have mastered. For example, your dog already knows how to sit—she does this on her own. Simply start rewarding her for doing so. Watch for when she starts the action, give her the "sit" command, and when her tail makes contact with the floor, give her lots and lots of praise, pets, and a treat. Clicker training—a technique that uses a *click* to signal the dog that she's done something right—is a positive way to teach new behaviors at any age. Learning something new now and then helps keep her mental abilities sharp.

Choose a new route for your daily walk to add variety, new sounds and scents, to her world. Add a birdbath or squirrel feeder to the backyard, near the dog's favorite window, for viewing pleasure and entertainment. Even if she's no longer able to chase them, she'll be intrigued by their presence. If your dog enjoys the company of other dogs, talk to friends about setting up play dates for your pets to meet. Just be sure to supervise play so that your friend's exuberant youngster doesn't bowl over your more sedate older dog.

Exercising your dog's mind is the best gift you can give to each other, because it delays the aging process of the brain. Keeping her mind healthy keeps you connected, and strengthens the bond you already share.

Golden Moments: Feeling Important

Madelene Rutz of Eureka has been involved in dogs—showing, competing, and just loving them—for more than thirty-five years. Today she has a total of eleven dogs. Five of them are senior-citizen canines over the age of eight.

She believes maintaining their health during their early years makes a positive difference in how they age. "I also think a tremendous amount of love has a lot to do with it," says Madelene. Genetics and family trees also have an influence. For instance, eight-year-old Toby, a black Labrador, has lots of white on his face. She attributes part of this to the seizures he's suffered over the years. In contrast, twelve-year-old "huggy-bear" Mike, another black Lab, has very little white on his face.

With so many dogs, it's important to keep accurate records. "I keep a diary on my dogs," says Madelene, and she thinks all owners should do the same. "If I see something unusual and write it down, then I can look back later to see, Oh, Molly hurt her back on this date." That's particularly important information the veterinarian may need, she says. "I can tell them what happened on what day, how they acted, what I gave them. Pay very close attention to your dogs, because we're the ones who live with them; we're the ones who see them every single day."

As her dogs grow older, she's made few concessions to age. But she has noticed they're shorter on patience. "They want everything *right now*—to be fed, to go out. They don't want to wait for everybody else," she says. More than anything, Madelene says she "listens" to what her dogs want. For instance, Mike was very close to attaining his Utility title in obedience competition when he developed arthritis in his front foot. "I decided there's no reason to put him through this. He doesn't realize he's getting a degree; that's only for me," says Madelene.

The older dogs have decided they don't want to be outside as much anymore. All the dogs sleep inside. Madelene has provided bedding that even the younger dogs enjoy. "You can buy them ready-made from dog-supply places, but I find it's easiest to buy orthopedic foam sheets at Wal-Mart or Target, cut it to the right size, and cover with a sheet," says Madelene. That way the padding can be made to fit in crates or in her van, or a full size can be used for a couple of dogs to share. "The sheets are easy to wash, so it can be kept nice and clean and they all have something soft to lie on." Some of her dogs like to sleep on the floor, others prefer the foam, and a few sleep with Madelene. "Brook has always slept next to me; she's always by my side," says Madelene of the nine-year-old Doberman.

She also makes sure all the dogs, whatever their age, get regular exercise. For the older dogs, just walking works well. And for aging competition dogs like Mike, exercise and "work" also can help maintain the dog's emotional health.

"Make them feel important," says Madelene. "Make them feel they're just as important as the younger ones who are still working." For instance, although Mike isn't able to compete, she still has him go through some of the exercises. "That makes him still think he's doing his obedience and he's rewarded with his treats just like always," she says. Set the jumps low so the dog can succeed and not be hurt, but still feel like a winner. Throw the Frisbee so your dog doesn't have to leap to catch it. "Self-esteem is incredibly important," she says. "Mike doesn't have to compete with the other dogs. He's still just as happy as peaches that he's done his retrieving!"

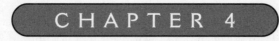

CHAPTER 4

Nursing Care

Dogs can live with illness and infirmity and still be happy. They don't worry about looking "funny" if they lose a leg to cancer—they're just ecstatic the pain went away. Exactly how to define a "good" quality of life varies between individual dogs and owners. How well or poorly a dog functions during illness or convalescence is influenced by veterinary support and your own care for them.

The greatest measure for quality of life is, Does he enjoy today? "When an owner questions what they should watch for, I suggest they write a list of things Jasper loves to do," says Laura Garret, DVM. Maybe he begs for a walk twice a day, or carries his ball everywhere. Then one day he sleeps through walk time. And the next week he has no interest in playing fetch. With chronic illnesses and aging in general, changes can be so gradual that owners don't see them, says Dr. Garret. Having a concrete list to look back on helps you measure these changes.

CARE CONSIDERATIONS

Old animals that are otherwise healthy may lose their sight or hearing, or develop other infirmities that require nothing more than a few environmental accommodations to keep them safe and comfortable. For the animals that do have a life-threatening problem, however, additional questions must be asked. How will treatment affect his condition? Is a cure possible? If not, will a given treatment stop or slow the progression of the condition, and for how long? Will it improve the way he feels, or make him feel worse? Is it worthwhile to make him feel worse for a short time to improve his longevity? Based on these answers, owners can then decide what care is best for their dog.

"Pets wake up every day and say, 'This is how I feel today,' " says Nicole Ehrhart, VMD, a cancer specialist and surgeon at the University of Illinois. "If we're making their treatment worse than their disease, even for long-term gain, the pet doesn't understand that." Many older dogs don't have a lot of time to waste feeling bad—every minute, every day counts when your German Shepherd is thirteen or your Yorkshire Terrier is seventeen. "You hate for them to spend the time they have left in the hospital," she says. "It's something you really have to weigh with an owner."

Based on these considerations, owners can choose (1) curative therapy—hard-hitting treatment that still keeps in mind quality of life; (2) palliative care—treatment to keep the dog comfortable when a cure isn't possible; or (3) hospice care.

"With the palliative realm you accept that the cancer [or other condition] will progress, that quality of life is now reasonable, and so we'll prevent symptoms as long as we possibly can," says Dr. Ehrhart. That might be the best choice for an old dog who is unable to survive radical surgery, for example, or for an animal whose cancer is far advanced. It may also be an economical or ethical choice for owners who aren't interested in aggressive treatment and just want to keep their dog comfortable during the time he has left. Palliative options often involve minimal cost and few hospitalizations when nursing care is provided at home, says Dr. Ehrhart.

Hospice is essentially end-of-life care. "It's where we say there's really nothing further we can do, this is progressing rapidly, we're losing the battle, and it's near the end," says Dr. Ehrhart. "Let's keep him comfortable at home."

PAIN MANAGEMENT

People who love their pets do not want them to suffer. They want them to be comfortable, come what may. Unfortunately, there is no objective way to evaluate pain in animals—they can't tell us, "That hurts" the way people do.

On top of that, Steven L. Marks, BVSc, says, "What you think is painful and what I think is painful may be different." One person thinks the dog is crying or howling because of pain and gives medicine, while someone else thinks he just wants attention—and talking and petting delivers the balm.

ANGEL'S GATE

In most cases, hospice for pets means the dog is made comfortable in the owner's home. Owners unable to care for their animals' end-of-life needs have few other options, but the hospice movement for pets is slowly gaining recognition. In early 2002, the American Veterinary Medical Association approved guidelines for animal hospice care, and today there are a handful of model pet hospices set up similarly to their human counterparts. Angel's Gate, founded nearly a decade ago by registered nurse Susan Marino and partner Victor LaBruna, was one of the first and is still the largest of its kind.

Angel's Gate (www.angelsgate.org) is a nonprofit animal-care facility where animals who are terminally ill, elderly, or physically challenged come to live out their days in peace, dignity, and love. Marino cares for cats, dogs, rabbits, horses, and critters of all kinds in her Long Island sanctuary. "Our focus is on wellness and quality of life," says Marino. "We provide for the physical, emotional, and spiritual needs of each animal with a holistic approach to caring."

Marino hopes that Angel's Gate will become a model for animal hospices all over the country. Currently she charges no fee for hospice care and relies on private donations to fund the cost of pet food, veterinary visits, acupuncture, massage, swim therapy, and other care options offered to maintain quality of life.

Not all pain is severe or sudden. Chronic pain is more typical in older dogs. Even the inflammation and discomfort of skin disease falls into the "pain" category, says William Tranquilli, DVM. "The long-acting steroid products given to reduce inflammation of the skin are a type of pain management," he says. Antibiotics that cure a sore throat by reducing an infection are addressing pain. The first sign of disease in people is often a complaint of pain. "Dogs can't say, 'I'm in pain'; they're waiting for the vet to find it," says Dr. Tranquilli. Whether pain arises from arthritis, a tumor, or sore skin, it's something to which owners and veterinarians must be sensitive.

In terms of major surgeries and the management of postoperative pain, Dr. Ehrhart says veterinary medicine has much to offer. "For example, oral-cavity cancers are really common in older dogs, and surgery may involve removing part of the jaw," she says. That sounds horrendous, and owners often fear putting their pet through such radical treatment. "But actually, animals recover from surgery like this extremely well," says Dr. Ehrhart. "There's extremely good cosmetic results, and we are able to very effectively manage postoperative pain." People are often surprised to see their dogs walking out of the hospital two days after surgery, feeling good and still able to eat.

"The degree to which we experience pain has a lot to do with fear," she says. A dog doesn't anticipate or think about tomorrow—he just wakes up and says, "this is how I feel today." "They don't worry about how long it's going to last, or how much worse it might get. We can make them feel decent every day, and they're happy."

Golden Moments: Kramer's Legacy

Janine and Barry Adams were first-time dog owners when Kramer, a black Standard Poodle, came into their lives. "Kramer is a fabulous dog, but he was clearly bred for his looks," says Janine. "He's very smart, but his health isn't very good. I'm sure there's a genetic component."

He was pretty healthy up until age six, and Janine says she took great pains providing all the recommended preventive veterinary care, such as annual vac-

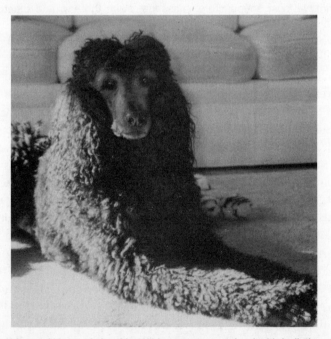

Many of Kramer's health problems were resolved with holistic treatments.   *(Photo Credit: Janine Adams)*

cinations. Today, aware of potential immune problems from overvaccination, Janine worries her diligence might have prompted some of Kramer's problems.

Nearly all of the dog's health concerns are autoimmune in origin—that is, caused by a malfunction of the immune system that attacks the dog's body. At age six, Kramer was hospitalized with dangerous gastrointestinal problems that were ultimately diagnosed as inflammatory bowel disease (IBD). The mechanism of this disease isn't completely understood, but it's thought to be linked to allergies in which the lining of the intestines becomes inflamed and interferes with the normal processing of food. IBD is typically treated with steroids to suppress the overreaction of the immune system, along with a change in diet.

Not long after that, Kramer was diagnosed with hypothyroidism. The thyroid gland regulates the metabolism, and hypothyroidism—a slowing down of body processes—results when not enough hormones are produced. Kramer's hypothyroidism is treated with an oral medication called seloxine.

"Then at seven, he was diagnosed with lupoid ochydystrophy," says Janine. "That's basically lupus [another autoimmune disease] affecting the nail beds—his toenails were falling off." On top of that, Kramer was diagnosed with Addison's disease when he was eight years old. The disease is caused by a malfunction of the adrenal glands; they don't produce enough cortisol. "He gets a DOCP shot every twenty-eight days to replace the aminoalacorticoid," says Janine, "and every other day he gets some hydrocortisone to replace the glucocorticoid. It's a little balancing act."

With so many different health problems, and various medications, Janine says it took a while to make everything work well together. "Once we got those things worked out, he was feeling much better."

But six weeks later, he had a life-threatening episode of bloat (gastric dilatation volvulus), in which the stomach fills with gas and may twist inside the body. "That may be the one nonautoimmune problem he's had," says Janine. Researchers are still seeking the causes of bloat, but Kramer fits the profile of predisposed dogs—middle-aged or older, large breed, deep-chested, and prone to stress. "Kramer's a little bit cautious and pessimistic, and very serious," says Janine.

As each new problem arose, Janine looked for ways of keeping Kramer as happy and healthy as possible. Her search ultimately led her to Dr. Conrad Kruesi, a holistic veterinarian in Vermont, who is a great believer in natural diets to improve pet health. Dr. Kruesi uses a biomedical microanalysis of the blood to pinpoint nutritional deficiencies and then make adjustments in the diet. Janine says the raw diet she feeds Kramer that was designed by Dr. Kruesi has made all the difference in the world. He also recommends appropriate supplements, vitamins and minerals for each animal's specific deficiencies. Kramer gets more than twenty pills a day, given in cream cheese. "He thinks it's swell," says Janine.

"I'm not a brave person when it comes to my dogs' health," adds Janine. "So I get very specific recommendations from Dr. Kruesi. I don't worry about screwing up and giving them an unbalanced diet, because he's checking it so carefully all the time."

At age nine, Kramer looks younger, feels better, and is healthier than since he was six. "This regimen is working beautifully for him," says Janine. "He's got energy and he's playing Frisbee and his nails are good, and all his lupus symptoms are gone. Kramer's a big Frisbee dog. He's not quite as good at catching them as he was when he was younger, but he still puts out a big effort. I couldn't be happier about it."

Janine and Barry made several lifestyle changes to accommodate their two aging dogs. Scout, a year younger than Kramer, was recently diagnosed with cancer. Stress could bring on another bloat attack for Kramer, and he's already more prone to stress because of his Addison's. If he was alone and he bloated again, he'd die. "So we made the commitment not to leave them alone," says Janine, who already works out of her home office. She says it really wasn't that difficult, but they did have to cancel some business trips and turn down a few invitations. They've also had to curtail Kramer's car trips, because he gets too excited.

They feed the dogs four times a day. Smaller, more frequent meals are thought to reduce the potential for bloat. Processing the protein in smaller amounts is also more helpful for Scout, who lost one kidney to the cancer.

Janine says having a partnership with your veterinarian, especially when your dog is older, is incredibly important. She keeps her own record of each dog's health reports. Kramer's are kept in three binders, each about three inches thick. "Get a copy of the animal's blood test results, because when you want to do research on your own it provides really valuable information," she advises.

It worries her that people often attribute behavior or health changes to "old age" when there might be other factors at work. "I really don't think of my dogs as old dogs, and they don't act like old dogs," she says. "I'm very aware of their health. But I choose to think in a positive way, to focus on their youth and not their age."

Janine says her world changed when Kramer joined her. "He turned our lives upside down because we were clueless dog owners," she says.

On December 3, 2001, Kramer was diagnosed with hemangiosarcoma, a cancer of the spleen and heart, and the Adamses opted for palliative care.

The brave boy passed away two days after Christmas, at home, in the company of the people he loved best.

Because of his influence, Janine says she learned new ways to deal with his problems, and she changed careers. Today she is an award-winning professional writer focused on dogs and their care. Kramer's legacy lives on in the lives of the dogs and people she touches through her work.

OWNER ATTENTION

Whether it involves hospitalization or home care, illness causes anxiety and stress. "If nobody visited you in the hospital for two weeks, you'd be depressed. So is your dog," says Sheila McCullough, DVM, an internist at the University of Illinois. Stress makes the immune system less efficient, and depression can cause loss of appetite and refusal to eat or move around. Regular owner visits improve the pet's attitude and make a positive difference in recovery, says Dr. McCullough.

It is also incredibly valuable to talk to other owners who have gone through a similar situation with their dog, says Dr. Garret. "Our clients start talking to each other in the waiting room. It's great!" Often pet owners feel isolated and may not always have the support or understanding of friends or family members. Talking with people with similar experiences validates their feelings. "They understand, because they've been through it too," says Dr. Garret. Other dog owners also can offer suggestions and advice for dealing with the situation.

Oftentimes your veterinarian will dispense medication for you to administer to your dog at home. During your lifetime together, it's likely you've already had experience giving a pill now and then, or putting drops in his ears.

Care for chronic problems, though, may demand more than you're accustomed to giving. Dogs recuperating from surgery with mobility problems may need your help walking, or being kept clean when they can't make it outside. Diseases such as diabetes or kidney failure may require injections or fluid therapy that can be administered much more economically at home, and with less stress to the dog.

Restraint

When dogs feel under the weather, their tempers may grow short even with a beloved owner. It's hard to tell him that you're "pilling" him for his own good, or that he must leave that sore alone or it won't heal. Struggling and getting upset won't help either his emotional or physical state. The best way to deal with treatments is to safely restrain your dog. This prevents either one of you from being accidentally hurt.

Your veterinarian can demonstrate how to use an effective restraint for your dog. Different techniques work best for small- to large-size dogs. Usually, an extra pair of hands makes medicating go much more smoothly. One of you restrains while the other medicates.

The restraint technique you choose should depend on which part of the body requires attention. For instance, a muzzle wouldn't be appropriate if you needed to treat a wound inside the mouth.

Here are some of the most common types of restraints.

- **Muzzle:** Frazzled doggy nerves or a painful touch may prompt the most loving dog to snap in reflex. A muzzle gently holds the dog's mouth closed so he can't bite. A variety of commercial muzzles are available from pet supply stores that fit large to small, sharp- to snub-nosed dogs. You can also make your own muzzle with a length of soft cloth, a strip of roll gauze, or even a length of panty hose. Tie a loop in the material and slip it over the dog's nose—you may need someone to help you steady his head. Snug the knot over the top of his nose, then bring the ends down underneath and tie a second knot below his chin. Finally, draw the ends back behind his neck and tie in a bow behind his ears.
- **Hug restraint:** Used to immobilize the abdomen, legs, chest, or back for treatment, the hug restraint works best on dogs over twenty pounds. Bring one arm under and around the dog's neck in a half-nelson posture, and hug. With the other arm, reach over and around his chest and pull him closer to your chest.
- **Reclining restraint:** This technique works particularly well on medium to large dogs. Place your dog on his side, with the treatment area facing up for easy access. Grasp the ankle of the foreleg that's nearest the ground while pressing your forearm across his shoulders to hold him gently down. Your other hand grasps the ankle of the hind leg that's against the ground while pressing that forearm across his hips.
- **Stretch restraint:** Small dogs may be restrained most easily against the tabletop or floor by grasping the loose skin at the back of the neck—scruff—with one hand. Capture both hind feet with the other hand. Then gently stretch him out flat. *Warning:* This restraint technique should *not* be used with dogs that have prominent eyes, like Pekingese.

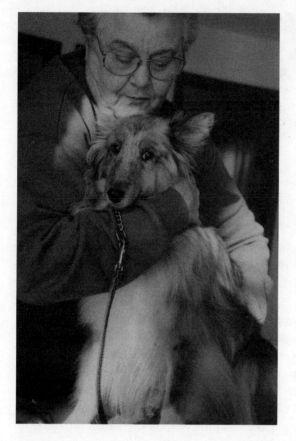

The hug restraint works well on medium and larger size dogs. *(Photo Credit: Amy D. Shojai)*

- **Kneeling restraint:** This is the best technique for Pekingese and other prominent-eyed dogs, because pressure around their necks may cause prolapsed eyeballs—the eyes pop out of the socket. Kneeling restraint also works very well on any small dog, especially when you must medicate by yourself. Place the dog on the floor between your knees, facing out. Then put one hand on top of the head, and the other beneath his jaw to hold him still.
- **Collar restraint:** Commercial cone-shaped collars that surround the pet's neck like the elaborate ruff of an Elizabethan noble are called Elizabethan collars or E-collars. They come in a variety of sizes to fit any pet. However, some dogs strenuously object to wearing these collars because they have trouble eating or navigating with them on. A newer alternative, called a Bite-Not Collar, is similar to the stiff cervical collars designed for people to wear after neck injuries. These collars are used to

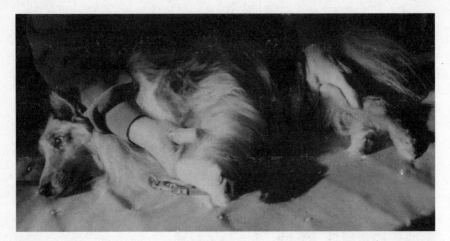

The reclining restraint is particularly helpful with dogs that are otherwise hard to control. It can be difficult to give oral medicine, though, when the dog is in this position. *(Photo Credit: Amy D. Shojai)*

prevent dogs from pawing head wounds or from chewing body injuries. They are available at most pet supply stores or from your veterinarian.

- **Body restraints:** Commercial products such as the WoundWear Body Suit have been developed to allow dogs freedom to move while keeping them from bothering healing wounds, stitches, stomach tubes, or catheters. A homemade body wrap can work just as well for short convalescence periods. To protect shoulder and chest areas, fit the dog with a T-shirt—his front legs go through the arms, his head through the neck, and the loose end is safety-pinned behind his rear legs beneath the tail. For body-area protection, stand your dog on a towel or sheet, mark the positions of his feet on the material, and cut out holes in these places. Then put him back on the cloth with his feet through the openings. Pull it up over his legs, and secure over his back with safety pins.

Medication

You may be required to give your dog a wide range of medications in a variety of forms. Often you can request that a pill be turned into a liquid, or compounded into a flavored treat. Some medicines can even be turned into a *transdermal* preparation that is smeared on and absorbed by the skin—no pilling necessary.

Medicine is designed to treat a particular condition or illness and help your dog feel better. If you have to fight your dog to get the medicine down, his quality of life may suffer and the bond you share may be damaged. Don't hesitate to ask your veterinarian for alternatives. After all, your dog's comfort—even his life—may be at stake.

- **Topical treatment:** Topical application—that is, on-the-skin treatment—usually comes as an ointment, salve, or spray. It is the easiest to administer. Some medicines for pain may come as a patch that's stuck onto a shaved area of the dog's body. Dogs often want to lick off the medicine or chew the patch. The biggest challenge you'll have is making sure your dog leaves the treatment alone long enough for it to work.
- **Liquid medicine:** Applicators similar to eyedroppers or needleless syringes often come with the medication. Liquid oral medicine is usually easier to give than pill forms. Draw up the prescribed amount and then tip your dog's head up toward the ceiling. Insert the tip of the applicator into the corner of the mouth, and squirt the medicine into his cheek, keeping his mouth closed. You may need to stroke his throat and keep his head tilted up until you see him swallow. If your veterinarian has given the okay, follow the medicine with a favorite treat. That leaves the dog with a good-tasting reward, and something to look forward to the next time around.
- **Pills**: Dogs often swallow pills more readily when they're hidden in a tasty lump of liverwurst or cheese. It's fine to "bribe" dogs to take their medicine as long as it doesn't interfere with the effectiveness of the drug—ask your veterinarian to be sure. However, sometimes dogs learn to swallow the treat and spit out the pill. You'll have to make sure he gets the real medicine or it won't do him any good.

    To pill your dog, circle the top of his muzzle with one hand, pressing his lips gently against his teeth just behind the large, pointed canine teeth. That prompts him to open wide, and when he does, push the pill to the back of his tongue with your other hand. If you fear for your fingers, use a pill syringe (pill gun or pill dispenser), a hollow plastic tube that places the pill at the back of his throat. Then close his mouth, and gently hold it closed while stroking his throat or gently blowing on his nose to induce him to swallow. Butter or margarine on the pill helps grease its trip down his throat. Most pets lick their nose after they swallow, so watch for this cue. Have a treat

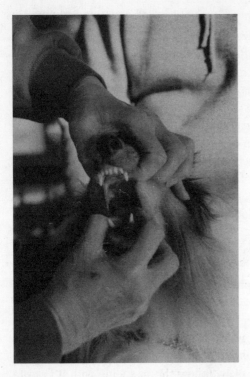

Place one hand over the top of the dog's muzzle and gently press his lips against the teeth. Generally that will prompt him to open wide, so that you can pop a pill inside with your other hand. *(Photo Credit: Amy D. Shojai)*

Generally it takes two people to handle the dog to administer eye medicine—one to restrain and the other to treat. *(Photo Credit: Amy D. Shojai)*

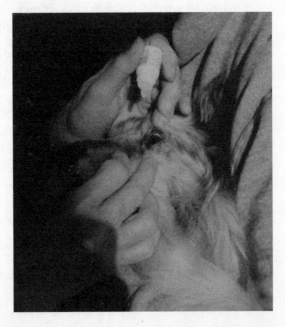

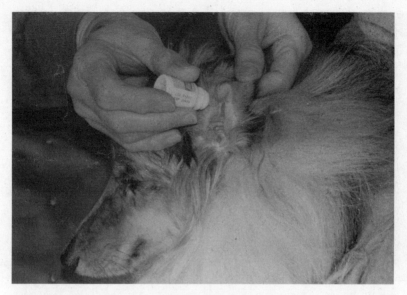

As long as the ears are not painful, most dogs don't mind having ear medicine applied at home.   *(Photo Credit: Amy D. Shojai)*

ready to immediately wash down the pill—some dogs forget to spit
out the medicine in favor of lapping up the treat.

- **Eye medicine:** Liquid and ointment medications are applied the same
  way to your dog's eyes. Point his head toward the ceiling, gently pull
  down the lower eyelid, and drip or squirt the recommended dosage
  into the cupped tissue. Then release the eyelid and allow your dog to
  blink, which spreads the medicine evenly over the surface of the eye.

- **Ear medicine:** The canine ear canal resembles an L, with the
  eardrum right at the foot of the L. Ear medicine is usually in liquid or
  ointment form so it's easier to get the medicine where it needs to go.
  Tip the dog's head so the opening of the affected ear is aimed at the
  ceiling. Place several drops of the medicine into the canal, while
  grasping the dog's earflap in a gentle but firm grip. That keeps him
  from immediately shaking his head and spraying the medicine everywhere. With your free hand, massage the base of the dog's ear, to
  help spread the medicine deeper into the canal. Dogs with itchy ears
  tend to enjoy this, and may moan and lean into the massage. But if
  the dog's ears are painful, a few treatments at the veterinarian may be
  required to get him to the point where he'll allow you to medicate
  him at home.

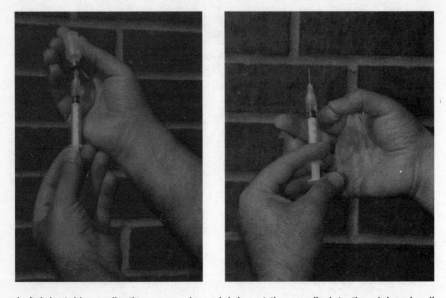

Left: Injectable medications come in a vial. Insert the needle into the vial and pull back on the plunger to fill the syringe to the prescribed level. Your veterinarian will explain exactly how much to give for each dose.   *(Photo Credit: Amy D. Shojai)*
Right: Once the syringe is filled, withdraw the needle from the vial and point it toward the ceiling. Thump the syringe once or twice to dislodge any air bubbles in the liquid—they'll rise to the end of the needle so you can carefully squeeze them out with the plunger.   *(Photo Credit: Amy D. Shojai)*

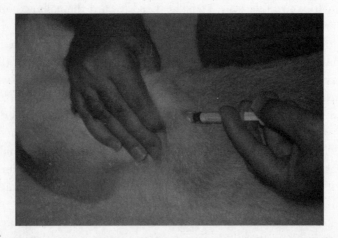

Grasp the loose skin over the dog's neck and shoulders to form a "tent" of the tissue. Insert the needle at the base of the tented skin, horizontal to the dog's body, then depress the plunger to administer the medication. Remove the needle and gently rub the exit.   *(Photo Credit: Amy D. Shojai)*

- **Injections:** Needles scare people much more than they do dogs. Giving the medicine by injection often provides quicker relief, and for certain conditions is the only option. For example, diabetic dogs typically require insulin shots. For an injection, draw up the specified amount of medication into the syringe. Point the needle at the ceiling and gently thump the syringe so any air bubbles float to the needle and can be squeezed out with slight pressure on the plunger. Watch for a small drop of fluid to appear out of the needle, which means the air is gone and you're ready to give the injection. Either kneel on the floor next to your dog or place him on a countertop. Grasp the loose skin over the shoulders with one hand, and insert the needle horizontally into the skin with the other. Depress the plunger, withdraw the needle, and briefly rub the spot to remove the sting and speed absorption.

COMFORT ZONE

Pill Pals are tiny feeding cubes made from hormone-free New Zealand beef, designed with a slit in the center. This allows room for a pill or capsule to be tucked inside, one option for bribing your dog to take his medicine. Pill Pals are available in a resealable foil pouch from Oceania Products, www.oceaniaproducts.com.

Fluid Therapy

Pets with chronic conditions such as kidney failure, liver disease, or intestinal problems often need ongoing fluid therapy on a daily basis. You can get the proper supplies from your veterinarian—an IV kit with a plastic line and a supply of large-gauge needles. Appropriate fluids might be saline for kidney disease, dextrose (sugar) solutions for nutritional support, or balanced electrolyte solutions. For routine fluid therapy, you won't be asked to give fluid into the veins because that requires special skills. Instead, you give the fluid under the dog's skin—subcutaneous or SubQ administration. Once your veterinarian demonstrates, it's easy to administer SubQ fluids to your pet at home.

1. Suspend the bag higher than the pet, so that gravity helps the fluid flow smoothly. A coat hanger hooked over the top of a door or cabinet can make a fine holder.
2. Spread a towel or favorite blanket on the floor or tabletop to create a

comfortable surface for your pet to lie down on. He'll need to stay still for up to twenty minutes. Ask the veterinarian if a heating pad placed underneath a couple of layers of blanket is a good idea. Otherwise, the fluids can be chilly for the pet.

3. Pets that need fluid therapy will have lots of loose skin, and you need to insert the needle so that the fluid drains into the space right under the loose tissue. Anywhere on the body will work, but the best location is often right between the shoulder blades or right above the ribs. Grasp the skin with one hand and "tent" it—draw it up off the solid muscle. Then press the sharp end of the needle firmly into the skin, between your hand that holds the flesh and the solid muscle of the pet's body. You'll need to push pretty hard, because the needle will be large and a pet's skin can be tough. Push in at a horizontal angle level with the body until you no longer see any of the needle, only the plastic head that houses the plastic IV line. Don't be surprised if the pet flinches a bit. Once the needle is in place, he should settle down and won't be much bothered by the therapy.

4. Once the needle is in place, let go of the tented skin and let it fall back into place. Open up the release valve on the plastic line, so that the fluid begins to drain down and into the needle. Watch the container of fluid until the full dosage has been given. A severely dehydrated pet may need 20 milliliters per pound, while for other conditions, 10 milliliters per pound once a day may be enough. As fluid runs into the skin, you'll see the skin start to balloon with liquid. This does not hurt the pet, although it may feel a bit cool, and will tend to settle and spread out under the skin. The fluid will be gradually absorbed into the body and the balloon will deflate.

5. Shut off the valve on the IV line to stop the fluid, and then gently remove the needle from your pet. It's normal for a small amount of fluid to leak back out of the injection site—especially when given over the shoulders. Giving fluid over the ribs with the needle inserted downward will reduce this loss. Massaging the area will help the injection site hole to close.

Nutritional Support

Good nutrition is vital to not only maintain the older dog's health, but also to support him during illness and help him recover. Old dogs have fewer nutritional reserves. While missing a meal or two probably wouldn't hurt a dog in his prime, it can be the turning point on a downhill slide for seniors.

COMFORT ZONE

Ask your veterinarian about the new "indwelling catheters" designed for subQ administration of fluid. Dr. Martin G. St. Germain of Practivet (www.practivet.com) developed the administration unit, called the Greta Implantable Fluid Tube (GIF-Tube). The nine-inch silicon tube is surgically implanted just beneath the pet's skin, and a small skirt of material is sutured in place to hold the tube steady. An injection port is attached to the outside portion of the tube. The veterinarian will change the port each month, but the tube itself can remain in place for up to a year. A needleless injector connects to administer fluids through the port. That allows you to give fluids to your dog without poking him with a needle.

Food refusal can be complicated by prescribed changes in diets due to chronic conditions, such as heart or kidney failure. While some breeds, especially hunting dogs, may eat anything that doesn't move faster than they do, Toy breeds are notoriously fussy about their food. Dogs that develop liver disease or other serious illnesses may refuse to eat anything at all. A number of techniques can help keep your dog eating well.

- **Switch foods slowly:** Nothing will upset the aging dog's tummy more quickly, or prompt him to snub the bowl with more determination, than an abrupt diet change. Because of aging changes to the dog's senses of smell and taste, changing a food allegiance can be tough because he's "trained" his taste buds to recognize and prefer the same food, says Nancy E. Rawson, Ph.D., an expert on taste and smell sense in pets. If a switch is in order—whether to a quality "senior" product or a therapeutic diet for a health condition—do so gradually. Offer a 50/50 mixture of the new diet with the old food for the first week. Then give him a third of the old mixed with two-thirds of new food for another several days, and finally feed the new food exclusively.

- **Offer alternatives:** Remember, no matter how great a new diet may be, it does no good until it moves out of the bowl and into your dog. Help him learn to love it. But if he still refuses after the gradual switch, ask your veterinarian about comparable alternatives. Several pet food companies offer lines of therapeutic foods, and your dog may prefer one brand over another.

- **Soften the food:** This is particularly helpful for aged dogs with painful teeth or mouths. Dogs don't tend to chew their food, and large or hard kibble can be difficult to manage for senior dogs. Change to a canned or soft-moist formula, or soften the dry diet by adding a cup of water for every cup of dry food. Avoid milk; that gives some dogs diarrhea and gas.

- **Increase the smell:** Scent is incredibly important to dogs. Palatability of the food is dictated not only by taste and mouth feel, but also by smell. You may be able to spark his appetite by making the food more pungent. Try adding warm water or an unsalted chicken broth drizzle over the food, and heating in the microwave for a few seconds. The warmth unlocks the aroma and the temperature may also help tempt the appetite.
- **Feed more frequent, smaller meals:** Don't expect the dog to gulp down the entire bowl the way he did in his youth. Offer a serving for twenty minutes, then give the dog's nose and taste buds a chance to rest for thirty to sixty minutes. That allows the chemical sensory pathways in the nose and tongue to "reset," says Dr. Rawson, and helps them better detect how yummy the food is.
- **Tube feeding:** Chronic-care and critical-care patients that refuse to eat for two or three days are candidates for tube feeding. It's nearly impossible to force-feed an adult dog, even when they're weakened from illness. However, oftentimes dogs are more likely to eat for an owner than they are in the hospital surrounded by strange people, sights, and smells.

  The most effective way to get nutrition into these dogs is to place a tube into the stomach through which a soft diet can be fed. This requires anesthesia. One end of the large-bore flexible gastrotomy tube opens into the dog's stomach, while the other exits through the abdominal wall at his side. The tube makes it possible to feed the animal for weeks or months. Usually, a high-calorie soft diet is fed one syringeful at a time, and can be managed by the owner at home.

Wound and Bandage Maintenance

Any wound from injury or surgery is subject to infection from the contamination of bacteria. Foreign material that infects wounds or bandages thrives in moist, warm environments. Therefore, the best defense against complications is keeping wounds and bandages clean and dry.

- **Clean the area:** Most times, the injured area will have been shaved and cleaned by the veterinarian. You'll just need to monitor the site for discharge, heat, or swelling—any of which may point to infection. The best way to clean a wound with the least amount of discomfort to your dog is using a cool-water flush to float out debris. Your hands never have to touch the area, which can be very tender. Your veterinarian may provide you with a cleansing solution, such as the non-stinging antiseptic Betadine Solution. Dilute this 50/50 with distilled water to the color of weak tea. Put the diluted Betadine Solution in a new plant sprayer, and spray the wound site to disinfect. Pat dry with gauze pads or a clean, lint-free cloth.

FEEDING FOR HEALTH

Getting concentrated and highly palatable nutrition quickly into the sick dog makes a big difference in how quickly he recovers. Most "recovery" type foods are available only through veterinarians. Examples include:

- Eukanuba Veterinary Diets, Nutritional Stress/Weight Gain Formula, Maximum-Calorie
- Hill's Prescription Diet Canine a/d or p/d
- IVD Select Care Canine Development Formula
- Waltham Canine Convalescence Support Diets
- Waltham Feline/Canine Rehydration Support (a glucose-electrolyte drink to help counter mild to moderate dehydration)

- **Protect the bandage:** A variety of bandages are designed for different injuries, and your veterinarian will show you how to change them, if necessary. Primarily, your job is to keep the bandage clean and dry. That can be a challenge, since most dogs go outside to eliminate, where they're exposed to dirt and rain. Cover the bandage with plastic to temporarily protect the area from the elements. A plastic bread wrapper or newspaper bag, for instance, can slip over a bandaged leg. Plastic wrap also works well, especially for body bandages. Plastic wrap sticks to itself but not to fur, and helps keep dirt and rain away from the injury.
- **Prevent canine chewing:** It's hard to explain to your dog why he shouldn't lick the sore or chew off the bandage. A collar restraint prevents the wrong kind of attention. It is also helpful to keep the dog occupied with a game or treat until the cleansed wound dries or the medicine is absorbed. You can often repel canine licking of suture sites or bandages by applying strong-smelling Vicks VapoRub next to

the incision or directly on bandages. The menthol tends to be off-putting. When a dog has ignored his bandage and then suddenly decides it must come off, ask your veterinarian to check the situation. Such sudden attention is almost always a sign of either infection underneath or a bandage that's too tight.

Providing nursing care for your dog at home can be a loving and meaningful experience for you both. In addition, it's helpful for you to be involved in his care, so you better understand his health situation.

"I strongly believe that owners need to participate in the care of a sick pet," says Dr. McCullough. Such participation may be as simple as visiting the pet in ICU each day, or as involved as performing actual nursing care at home.

Dogs recognize who and what they are connected with. When they see you visiting the hospital every day, or caring for their needs at home, they will respond more positively to treatment. "They know that protection is coming, that security is coming, that my owner/companion is here," says Dr. McCullough. "The pet really needs that kind of commitment."

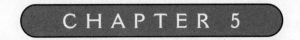

CHAPTER 5

Advanced-Care Options

According to the American Animal Hospital Association, 84 percent of owners surveyed said they refer to themselves as their pet's "mom" or "dad," and 74 percent would go into debt for their pet's well-being. Because so many of us consider dogs to be part of the family, we want to prolong that relationship for as long as possible. To do that, more and more owners seek a very high level of care, thereby spurring veterinary medicine to ever greater heights to answer the demand.

Your general-practice veterinarian has all the training and skills necessary to care for your dog throughout a healthy old age. However, specific health problems in geriatric dogs often benefit from the expertise of a veterinary specialist.

VETERINARY SPECIALISTS

After eight to ten years of study to attain their DVM or VMD (general practitioner's degree), veterinarians can continue with three to seven or more years of further study to qualify as "board-certified specialists" in a particular health discipline. There are more than twenty specialty boards, referred to as "colleges," which provide certification. A veterinary specialist is said to be a "diplomate" of a particular college specialty. The designation for a surgeon, for instance, would be Dr. Harry Smith, DVM, DACVS, which stands for diplomate, American College of Veterinary Surgeons.

Veterinary specialists typically have available a wider range of equipment, such as ultrasound and MRI (magnetic resonance imaging) for diagnosing and managing senior-dog health problems. Specialized equipment and treatment techniques are often too expensive for a local veterinary office to afford. Therefore, most advanced treatments are available only at veterinary teaching schools—there are twenty-seven in the United States—or at multidiscipline specialty practices, which are usually located in larger cities. Oftentimes, mobile practices bring specialists and their advanced technology, such as cardiac Doppler ultrasound and orthopedic surgery, to the general practitioner's office.

The specialist's training provides them with the skills necessary to perform advanced surgical techniques and treatment, from hip replacement and kidney dialysis to chemotherapy and cataract surgery. You will find the same kinds of specialists in veterinary medicine as those who practice in human specialty medicine.

SPECIALTIES FOR AGING DOGS

- Behaviorists (American College of Veterinary Behaviorists, or ACVB)
- Dentists (American Veterinary Dental College, or AVDC)
- Diagnostic imaging specialists, including cancer radiologists (American College of Veterinary Radiology, or ACVR)
- Eye specialists (American College of Veterinary Ophthalmologists, or ACVO)
- Internists, including cardiologists, neurologists, and cancer specialists (American College of Veterinary Internal Medicine, or ACVIM)
- Nutritionists (American College of Veterinary Nutrition, or ACVN)
- Skin specialists (American College of Veterinary Dermatology, or ACVD)
- Surgeons (American College of Veterinary Surgeons, or ACVS)

There are currently only three certifications available in complementary alternative veterinary medicine: acupuncture, chiropractic, and homeopathy. Physical therapy is also considered an alternative treatment by veterinary medicine, although it's long been a standard part of human medicine. "A new certification program in physical therapy was just started at the University of Tennessee," says Signe Beebe, DVM. The American Holistic Veterinary Medical Association out of Maryland provides a list of qualified complementary alternative practitioners on their Web site at www.ahvma.com.

People now recognize that veterinarians are physicians practicing in a medical field, and consider the veterinary specialist to be comparable to their situation when referred by a general practitioner. "In fact, it's very common for people to say, 'I wish my grandmother had gotten the care that you're providing for my dog,' " says Steven L. Marks, BVSc.

There are a few differences, though, that you might not expect. "People have no problem calling me at three o'clock in the morning, which they would never do with their physician, even for their child!" says Dr. Marks. This happens whether or not a twenty-four-hour veterinary emergency clinic is available. The strong correlation between human and veterinary medicine also has some negative effects when a human family member's medical experience has been less than pleasant. "When I say *chemotherapy*, they say, 'Oh, no!' We have to explain that in dogs the treatment is different," says Dr. Marks. For instance, dogs treated with chemotherapy don't lose their fur, and rarely suffer the side effects common to human chemotherapy. "The quality of medicine now is incredible. We can do some incredible things to improve quality of life," says Dr. Marks.

Specialty care tends to be more costly, just as it is in human medicine. In cases where finances are an issue, ask your veterinarian about other options. Universities may be seeking candidates for participation in reduced-cost experimental trials, or they may offer deferred-payment plans. And even though a Rolls-Royce chemotherapeutic drug or hip replacement surgery may be ideal, a Volkswagen therapy that's more affordable is nearly always available and may, in fact, offer very similar results. Cancer therapies and surgery, for example, can be expensive, while diet changes usually are much less costly. Whatever choice you make should take into account not only your pet's welfare, but also the size of your wallet.

GERIATRIC RESEARCH

Research is an evolutionary process. Canine geriatric research is particularly daunting because it requires large numbers of dogs to study over a great many years. This is very expensive, and finding large populations of old research animals is nearly impossible. Usually, veterinarians must rely on recruiting the owners of aging pet dogs to participate in studies. The exception is some large commercial pet food companies that maintain their own colonies of dogs used to help answer questions about canine nutrition and its impact on the dog's health.

Veterinary medicine is not static. The breakthroughs of the past become old news as more advanced information comes to light. Sometimes accepted wisdom is proved to be wrong, while other times new research builds on existing information for a greater understanding. In addition, veterinarians have found that some "old-fashioned" methods of treating disease, such as herbs, acupuncture, and nutritional supplements, offer incredible potential for maintaining quality of life, especially for the chronic care needs specific to senior dogs.

Conventional or Western medicine approaches, including surgery and state-of-the-art diagnostic tools, combined with alternative therapies, offer the best of all worlds, says Dr. Beebe. "Western medicine is very powerful and effective for certain things, such as surgery," she says. "You can't give herbs and acupuncture for that." Alternative approaches are often ideal for keeping the old dog feeling well during chronic illnesses. "Integrated medicine offers a greater chance of success because you're utilizing two very strong systems of medicine."

The American Animal Hospital's Pets and People Survey indicated that in 1999, about 30 percent of respondents were using some form of complementary or alternative veterinary medicine (CAVM) in caring for their pets. A survey of course and research programs among U.S. veterinary schools showed that seven of the twenty-seven veterinary schools had some educational program in CAVM. Eighty-seven percent of respondents believed that acupuncture, nutraceuticals (nutrition components used like drugs), nutritional supplements, and physical therapy should be included in the curriculum, and 61 percent indicated that herbal medicine should be included.

NUTRITION RESEARCH

Some people consider that the label "senior diet" is a marketing ploy. In years past, that may have been true. When senior diets were first developed about ten years ago, the focus was on reducing calories, based on the premise that older pets don't require as much energy. They aren't as active, many have been spayed or neutered, which may slightly decrease their metabolism, and often they're overweight.

Pet food companies created the first senior diet categories simply by replacing fat calories with fiber, says Sarah K. Abood, DVM. Protein levels were also reduced in these early formulations, because scientists believed this helped protect the aging dog's kidneys, says Dan Carey, DVM.

One of the biggest changes in the past three or four years lies in our understanding of protein requirements in aging dogs. "Dietary protein has absolutely no role in causing kidney disease, so there's no benefit to reducing protein for older dogs," says Dr. Carey. In fact, studies by many nutrition scientists indicate that older animals are at risk for developing other problems if they don't eat enough protein. The most recent research says aging dogs require at least the same levels of protein necessary to support growing puppies, says Dr. Abood.

Nutritional research also benefits the dental health of senior dogs, says Bill Gengler, DVM. Plaque is that scummy, slippery bacterial material that gets on our teeth and eventually crystallizes into calculus or tartar. Once calculus mineralizes, it cannot be brushed away—it must be scaled away with dental instruments. "If we can prevent or at least delay this biofilm from crystallizing, we have more opportunity for it to be brushed away or worn away by chewing," says Dr. Gengler. Sodium hexametaphosphate (sodium HMP) helps prevent crystals from forming and can now be found in some dog foods, treats, chew biscuits, and rawhides. Another innovation involves a woven edible fiber that's part of the biscuit. "It doesn't break apart as quickly, so the tooth goes in and out of it several times," says Dr. Gengler. "That has a mechanical abrading or scrubbing activity."

Food Restriction

One of the longest ongoing canine longevity studies, conducted by Nestlé Purina, began fourteen years ago with six-week-old Labrador Retriever puppies. Based on studies in many species (especially rodents), food restriction is the only known nutritional change that extends longevity, says Dottie LaFlamme, DVM. Primates are currently being studied, and the Nestlé Purina research looked at the effect food restriction might have on dogs over their natural lifetime.

The study involved forty-eight puppies. Littermates were chosen to remove as much genetic influence as possible. Puppies were divided into two groups, with twenty-four pups in each group, and each group was fed the exact same diet. "But for their entire life one group got 25 percent less [food] than the other group," says Dr. LaFlamme.

One of the very earliest observed effects was a significant reduction in orthopedic problems, says Dr. LaFlamme. There was a reduction in hip dysplasia and hip-joint laxity, and a reduction in arthritis both in the hip and in multiple joints. Orthopedic problems are a major risk with large-breed dogs, so this benefit has a pronounced effect on quality of life. Study results proved that keeping dogs lean can extend their life span by 15 percent—or nearly two years for the dogs in the study.

Antioxidants—Vitamin Age-Protection

"The big thing that's come along in the last couple years is the antioxidant story," says Dr. Carey. He says that by using the correct blend of antioxidants, you can actually reverse some age-related damage and give dogs the immune function of a much younger animal.

"The antioxidants are certain vitamins that protect the body against oxidation, which is the metabolic version of rust," says Dr. Carey. Our bodies use oxygen to help release energy. By breathing, we constantly bathe our tissues in oxygen, and oxidation by-products are responsible for damage to the tissues. Healthy animals are able to control this process so that the negative effects of oxidation are kept in check. "But the ability to manage those normal processes wanes," says Dr. Carey. Over time, the balance tends to tip toward increased oxidation, which speeds tissue damage, puts a damper on the immune system, and increases the affects of aging.

By giving the dog the right combination of vitamins, the oxidation process is put back in balance and aging is slowed, says Dr. Carey. In the right doses, vitamin E and beta carotene help slow aging, but too much loses this antioxidant effect. "If we have somewhere between 18 to 20 milligrams per kilogram of food, beta carotene will improve antibody response in aging dogs," says Dr. Carey.

Another vitamin, lutein, helps certain "scavenger" immune cells to maintain their ability to replicate. Maintaining a healthy population of these cells will allow invaders to be recognized and destroyed, says Dr. Carey.

Influencing the immune system using diet is another frontier for research, says Dr. Abood. Experimental diets in rats actually lessened the severity of age-related hearing loss, and William W. Ruehl, VMD, DACVP, says antioxidants may also prove useful in treating or even preventing age-related cataracts in dogs.

"We're going to see research just explode," says Dr. Abood. She predicts that as pet food companies make formulation decisions based on new discoveries about what's good for senior-dog health, they'll also apply this research to puppy foods and adult maintenance diets. That may blur the differences between regular adult dog foods and senior formulations. "If they're otherwise normal and healthy, [senior dogs] could stay on this adult maintenance food," says Dr. Abood.

Antioxidants may also help protect against cancers, especially those associated with damaged DNA. Early studies seem to suggest that antioxidants protect against DNA damage, says Dr. Carey, but it's still too early in the research to say for sure.

BRAIN RESEARCH

It follows that the proper mix of antioxidants and nutrition would also protect the brain, and keep dogs "thinking" young—therefore acting youthful—well into their golden years. An experimental diet developed by Hills does just that, says Blake Hawley, DVM. It contains very specific antioxidants, along with other nutrients such as folic acid and L-carnitine that protect against free-radical damage. "They actually promote mitochondrial health and improve energy metabolism," he says. In addition, specialized fatty acids (VHA and EPA) support membrane health in these neurons, along with specific carotenoids and flavonoids that come from natural fruit and vegetable sources that help scavenge free radicals to slow the oxidation process that promotes aging.

Studies of the aging dog brain are under way at the University of Toronto and the University of New Mexico. "We've also been collaborating with Carl W. Cotman, Ph.D., at the University of California Institute for Brain Aging and Dementia," says Norton William Milgram, Ph.D., a professor of pharmacology at the University of Toronto. Studies look at brain pathology to find out what happens to the brain and how it changes when dogs become quite old.

Dr. Milgram's team measured the age-related mental dysfunction and resulting behaviors of two groups of dogs when fed an experimental diet compared to a "regular" senior food. They hypothesized that a food enriched with antioxidants and mitochondrial enzymes should either slow down or partially reverse the changes in the brain that occur during aging.

The Toronto study began in 1998 with forty-eight Beagles aged ten to thirteen years old. The first year, each was evaluated to ensure they were equal in regards to physical and cognitive status. Half the dogs in the study received the experimental diet, and the other half got a regular commercial senior food. In addition, half of the dogs in each of the two groups led a "kennel" existence. But twelve dogs in each group were given "cognitive enrichment" each day.

The enrichment included a group of tests that measured the specific cognitive functions in dogs that are known to deteriorate with age. These include spatial ability and visual spatial memory—the ability to use environmental landmarks to navigate, and the ability to remember how to find their way. The tests also measured the dogs' ability to learn to solve relatively complicated problems, and tested their activity level, curiosity, and how they interact with people. "We tested these animals five days a week and gave them new problems to solve to make them use their brains," says Dr. Milgram. "Half the animals that were in controls and half in the diet group had this cognitive enrichment. That went on for a year."

Dr. Milgram ran a parallel study with young dogs aged three to five years old. "We didn't see any effect in diet in the young dogs, but we didn't expect to," he says. But in the ten- to thirteen-year-old dogs, those fed the experimental diet for as little as one month showed significant performance improvement on cognitive tests as compared to those on the regular diet. There was an even greater difference after they ate the special food for six months, and additional improvement at the one-year mark of the study.

Just the special diet alone helped, says Dr. Milgram, but the dogs that also were asked to "exercise" their brain with problem-solving five days a week for a year tested with the greatest cognitive ability of all. "These animals remain alert, and we're not seeing the rapid deterioration among the animals that we normally would have seen," he explains. To date, information about Dr. Milgram's study is available at www.beagle.scar.utoronto.ca/dacp.

More recently, the diet went through an in-home test by pet owners who were kept in the dark about the diet's purpose. After feeding the food, they reported improved interaction with their dogs, said their dogs had increased energy, reported 74 percent fewer housetraining accidents, and said that dogs enjoyed a higher quality of life. The new product, called Hill's Prescription Diet b/d (behavior diet), has just been made available through veterinarians. "It's not quite a fountain of youth but is quite dramatic," says Dr. Hawley.

COMFORT ZONE

Dogs with cognitive disorders often "forget" their housetraining. DuPont offers the Spillnet barrier to place between the carpet and the padding to protect the floor and prevent accumulated scents from housetraining accidents. The product is $2.50 to $3 per square yard. Contact www.stainmaster.com.

DRUG RESEARCH

New drugs become available all the time, and those designed for treating old-pet health concerns are at the forefront of veterinary research. For instance, research by Dr. David S. Bruyette and others regarding deprenyl, also known as selegiline, showed that dogs that received the drug daily over a six-month period aged less than dogs that didn't receive the drug. Today, the drug (brand name Anipryl) is prescribed for dogs suffering from cognitive disorders to help reverse the signs of canine senility. Interestingly, this drug is also used to treat the symptoms of Parkinson's disease in people.

Another example is heart medications used to treat common aging-heart conditions. ACE inhibitors (angiotension-converting enzyme), such as Atenolol, block nerve receptors on the heart and blood vessels to correct the irregular heartbeat caused by disease. People with heart problems also may take ACE inhibitors.

In fact, research, testing, and approval of new medicines take a long time and cost a lot, and some never reach veterinary approval. Medications that might also have application for human health concerns typically receive the most research funding. Therefore, veterinary medicine commonly "borrows" from the human health side to offer a wider range of treatment options to aging dogs. This is called "off-label" use and is perfectly acceptable as long as the pet owner is informed. A drug does not necessarily need to be officially approved for veterinary use. Many are not approved because testing takes so long and is cost prohibitive. Cancer drugs for dogs are almost always the same ones used in human chemotherapy treatments, as are most intravenous fluids and many of the pain medications.

"Veterinary medicine without human drugs would be like that old Beatles song—*only half the man he used to be*," says Nicholas Dodman, BVMS. "We have permission from the FDA to prescribe [human drugs] for cases where we think it's needed." The veterinarian must explain to the owner that the drug is being used off-label and is not licensed for use in dogs, although often its safety and usefulness have been confirmed by experience. "We can tell them how it will help their dog, what the side effects are, and that we're on the right side of the law," says Dr. Dodman.

Herbal Options

"Herbs are very good at helping stabilize the failing systems," says Dr. Beebe. "Chinese herbal medicine is really good for geriatric animals because it has minimal side effects." Old dogs that already suffer from failing kidneys or liver, for example, have greater difficulty handling the more powerful Western drugs. "That doesn't mean Western drugs are bad," she says. Holistic veterinarians say animals benefit twice from the right herbal medicine because herbs not only treat the problem, but also have the ability to strengthen ailing systems.

Very few herbs have been tested for safety or efficacy, and only a handful have any sort of FDA endorsement. In effect, one could say that *all* herbs are used off-label, and the best ones for canine health care have been proved by the test of time.

There is a very large margin of safety with the majority of herbs. But herbs are not benign. "If they were benign, they wouldn't be causing an effect, and what good would they be?" says Dr. Beebe.

Just because an herb is "natural" does not mean it is safe. For example, digitalis is a common heart-stimulating drug derived from the highly toxic foxglove plant. An herbal remedy for heart trouble is hawthorn (*Crataegus laevigata*). If both hawthorn and digitalis are given together, they can amplify each other's effects and cause an overdose reaction.

Another potential problem is that herbs are not regulated in the same way as commercial drugs. Different manufacturers may offer the same herb products but in very different strengths, although labeled identically. Some consumer investigations into "natural" products suggest that without regulation, it's difficult to be sure the ingredients on the label are really in the bottle. Therefore, before choosing an herbal treatment it's even more important to enlist the aid of a veterinarian who is knowledgeable in their use, of their interactions with other drugs, of the reputation of various manufacturers, and of the individual animal's medical history.

Pain Management

In the past, pain in dogs was discounted as minimal compared to human discomfort, or it was considered a necessary evil and useful to keep the dog from further injuring himself. Veterinarians and pet owners now recognize that dogs do experience similar pain, even though they may express it differently than people do. Managing pain effectively and humanely is not only an ethical issue; it also strikes at the heart of maintaining a good quality of life for aging dogs.

There has been an evolution in the theory of pet pain management. Pet pain is now considered a treatable ailment, whereas in the past it was rarely addressed at all. This interest has spurred drug companies to develop safe, effective pain medications for dogs. Today, a variety of canine analgesics are available, designed to alleviate specific kinds of discomfort.

"The biggest example is the arthritis issue," says William Tranquilli, DVM. Etogesic and Rimadyl are two of the newest NSAIDs (nonsteroidal anti-inflammatory drugs) approved specifically to address arthritis pain in dogs. "Meloxicam is really popular in Europe and Canada, and I think it will probably be coming to the States in the near future," says Dr. Tranquilli.

The Companion Animal Pain Management Consortium, launched in early 2001, was established to study and better understand the mechanisms and treatment of pain. Pfizer Animal Health supported the development of regional "pain centers," created at each of the veterinary schools at University of Tennessee, University of Illinois, and Colorado State University. "Here at Illinois, we have established a hospital pain team," says Dr. Tranquilli. Veterinary medicine is often so species- or specialty-oriented, the opportunity to benefit from other disciplines may not be easily achieved. The expertise of the critical care, oncology, orthopedics, anesthesiology, and ophthalmology faculties have been pooled to deal with chronic and acute pain syndromes in various ways. Treating chronic pain in dogs can sometimes provide insight into how to treat chronic pain in horses, for example.

Eventually, the consortium hopes to gather pertinent information into a formalized pain-management program that can be shared with other universities and large referral practices, and at veterinary conferences. It is hoped that pain management may someday become a specialty of its own. "Just like we have pain physicians, maybe we can have a pain veterinarian," says Dr. Tranquilli.

Chronic pain is addressed more often in senior dogs now than ever before. One of the best ways to keep track of your dog's discomfort is to observe and record how the dog acts before and after medication is given. Some behavior changes are so subtle you must pay close attention. For instance, how many times did your dog ask to go outside to play or relieve himself before the medicine? Asking to go out more often or willingly navigating the stairs are good measures of pain reduction for an arthritic dog. "We encourage pet owners to pay attention to what's going on, on a daily basis, so they can see if there's improvement with medication," says Dr. Tranquilli.

Acupuncture

Acupuncture, an ancient method of relieving pain without the side effects of drugs, is now an integral part of veterinary medicine endorsed by the American Veterinary Medical Association, says Dr. Beebe. Veterinarians are certified by IVAS, the International Veterinary Acupuncture Society, or by the American Academy of Veterinary Acupuncture (AAVA), to ensure that they have the proper training for animals.

COMFORT ZONE

Harp music has been used in human medicine, particularly in hospice situations, to alleviate pain and distress. Susan Raimond, an author, music therapist, and concert violinist and harpist, lectures with the International Harp Therapy Faculty in Richmond, Virginia. She has been a pioneer in harp therapy for animals.

Music, especially from the harp, will lower heart rate and blood pressure, slow respiration, increase endorphin levels (natural pain-control factors produced in the brain), and possibly increase longevity. Add harp music to your pet's environment as a stress reliever and pain modulator, or simply to improve his quality of life. It will help you feel better, too!

Acupuncture, in which long, thin needles are inserted into the body, has been used for several thousand years to successfully treat a wide range of health problems in both people and animals. "All the mechanisms of acupuncture are not understood," says Dr. Beebe. Traditional Chinese Medicine (TCM) says we are kept healthy by an energy flow called *qi* (pronounced "chee") that moves along specified pathways (meridians) throughout the body. The meridians connect to all the organs, skin, muscles, and nerves, and illness is described as an interruption or imbalance of this natural flow. Acupuncture corrects the imbalance and returns the dog (or person) to health by stimulating specific points found throughout the body along the meridians. Each point is associated with a particular body system.

This sounds very strange to Western ears. We're used to offering a drug to slow down or speed up the heart, rather than sticking a needle in a dog's ear. But modern diagnostic tests actually prove that a needle inserted in one part of the body does have an affect on other areas.

Certain parts of the brain light up during acupuncture, when measured using an MRI. For example, needling the outside of the foot (the part associated with the eyes) causes the same reaction in the brain as if the eyes actually saw a flash of light. "Stimulating specific points on the body can cause the release of certain chemical factors in the blood," says Dr. Beebe. Studies have shown that acupuncture stimulates the release of natural painkillers called endorphins, can reduce nausea, and can even affect heart rate and blood pressure.

"Acupuncture and herbs, the two mainstays of Traditional Chinese Medicine, work together to achieve healing in the elderly dog by improving the homeostasis of the body, rebalancing it, and helping to stabilize and slow down the degeneration of body systems," says Dr. Beebe. Holistic veterinarians believe acupuncture helps the body heal itself by stimulating circulation, relieving pain, and improving organ function, especially the failing organs of older animals. "Most of these holistic systems have been around for several thousand years, while Western medicine has been around for one hundred and fifty years," says Dr. Beebe. "There doesn't have to be a choice between them. A good doctor always offers all the options."

Golden Moments: Loving Andy

Gina Spadafori first noticed Andy had a little bit of a limp when the Shetland Sheepdog was about seven years old. "We have a couple real good orthopedic surgeons here in Sacramento, so I took him in to see if there was a problem with his hip. There was," says Gina. X rays showed early signs of arthritis. "At that time we put him on a buffered aspirin for his bad days."

The pretty tri-merle-and-tan dog became progressively worse over the years. Andy turned fifteen this past June, and now he's also got arthritis in his shoulder. "It wasn't really bad until the last two years," says Gina. "He's so smart, he's learned to compensate. He can do a little shimmy-hop and get up."

Andy has benefited from taking the nutraceuticals glucosamine and chondroitin, along with the arthritis medicine Rimadyl. There was a little bit of improvement followed by a leveling-off, says Gina, and the dog seemed to maintain a fairly consistent mobility and quality of life.

Then Andy went into a decline, and looked more uncomfortable. "He just could not get up. He'd try and give up, and try and give up, until eventually he managed it. But it hurt him," says Gina. "It was heartbreaking. I thought he wouldn't make it through the winter."

A friend recommended that she try acupuncture. Gina knew that it

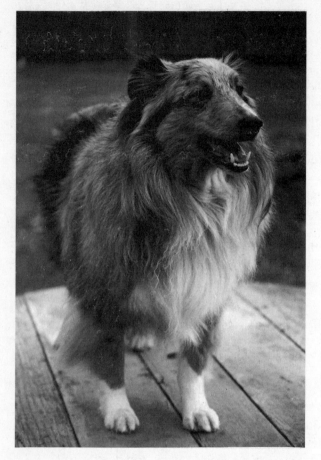

Acupuncture treatment along with herbal therapy helped keep Andy mobile when his arthritis acted up. *(Photo Credit: Gina Spadafori)*

wouldn't hurt Andy, and just might help make him more comfortable. Money wasn't an issue. "I spare no expense with my dogs," says Gina. But at this point, she had a very specific idea of what she wanted for Andy—anything that would make him feel better, but nothing invasive. "When I can't make him feel better anymore, he'll be euthanized."

She took her dog in for an evaluation with Dr. Signe Beebe, a certified veterinary acupuncturist and herbologist practicing at Sacramento Veterinary Surgical Services. Gina liked the idea that Dr. Beebe practiced complementary medicine along with input from cardiologists, surgeons, and other specialists. Andy would benefit from the best of all worlds.

"Gina's dog came in and had some significant osteoarthritis," says Dr. Beebe. The evaluation included both a Chinese and a Western exam, blood work, and X rays to help choose the most appropriate acupuncture points.

"You could see on the X rays that it was pretty darn obvious Andy was very arthritic," says Gina. As a complement, an herbal formula was also prescribed to help support his immune system.

The evaluation lasted about forty minutes; then Dr. Beebe reviewed the tests with the other veterinarians in the practice. Gina already knew about Andy's "old dog" heart murmur, a fairly mild problem the cardiologist considered consistent with his age. "He also has a lot of benign cysts; again that's in line with a fifteen-year-old dog," says Gina.

The next day Gina and Andy returned for the dog's first acupuncture treatment. Saline solution was injected into selected points around the joints of shoulders, hips, and knees. The entire session took about ten minutes.

During the treatment Dr. Beebe gave Andy lots of healthy treats, so the dog would associate the acupuncture with good things. "He's very agreeable, and Andy's a chowhound, so that works for him. He was in no discomfort at any point," says Gina.

The very next day Gina noticed an immediate improvement. She says Andy has maintained about a 10 to 15 percent improvement so far, after just three acupuncture treatments. Andy is also taking walks again, which will help loosen up his joints, improve circulation, and help flush toxins from his system. "So I take him for half a block out and half a block back, morning and night, even if it takes me forever to do it," says Gina.

Andy is feeling so much better he once again pays attention to his surroundings. "He'll pick up a toy and carry it to me. He wasn't doing that anymore, but now it's every day. And he's begging like crazy for treats when I'm eating. Before he didn't think it was worth bothering. Now he can find me and beg for treats."

Andy will continue with the acupuncture treatments for the time being, one every week or so, as needed. "He always used to be neutral on vet visits, but now he wants to go," says Gina. "He knows if he goes in *that* room, he gets cookies."

If the effects of the water acupuncture become less effective and he backslides, other levels of stimulation may give him more relief, such as mild electrostimulation using needles placed in the appropriate points.

People shouldn't consider some signs of aging as inevitable or incurable, says Gina. Treatments to make your dog feel better aren't necessarily that expensive, either. The herbs for Andy are about $16 a month, and the acupuncture sessions cost $55 per treatment. "Don't give up on your dog," says Gina. Andy clearly feels better, and that was Gina's goal all along.

SURGERY

Until relatively recently, treatments that required surgery were avoided in aging dogs, because many senior animals couldn't handle the anesthesia. Complications of heart disease, liver insufficiency, kidney failure, or other problems made anesthetic for even routine surgery a life-threatening risk.

Today, newer and safer anesthetics coupled with more accurate and noninvasive diagnostic tools such as Doppler ultrasound allow veterinarians to better choose the safest anesthetics and procedures for even the oldest dogs. Consequently, procedures such as dental surgeries and cataract repair are routinely performed on older dogs.

General-practice clinics are equipped to treat the older dog's arthritis with surgery, while specialty orthopedic surgeons may offer cutting-edge innovations. For instance, Dr. Mike Conzemius at Iowa State has developed total elbow replacement surgery for arthritic dogs. Cartilage transplant is another hot area, developed by Denver surgeon Dr. Robert Taylor, but is not yet widely available. Arthroscopy—noninvasive joint surgery using a specialized scope—reduces the amount of surgical injury to the joint so that dogs recover more quickly. This innovation is particularly important in older dogs that have less ability to bounce back from more invasive surgeries.

The most revolutionary and helpful surgeries are still very rare, and limited to only a handful of veterinary teaching universities. For example, acquired valvular heart disease is one of the most common killers of older dogs, and heart-valve replacement surgery to correct this problem is currently available only at Colorado State and University of Pennsylvania. Kidney transplantation for dogs with organ failure is limited to the University of California—Davis and a few other veterinary specialty centers.

Advanced care is more expensive and can be more difficult to find. But it is certainly available for those who request it. "I think we should not be afraid to offer the best care," says Jeff Johnson, DVM, a general practitioner with Four Paws Animal Hospital in Eagle River, Alaska. "A lot of times that's what people demand."

Not offering all the options shortchanges the veterinarian, the client— and the dog most of all, says Dr. Johnson. "It depends on what the client wants to do. It works best if the owner realizes what are the pros and cons, and what they're going to have to deal with [in terms of] home care."

Studies of canine longevity and aging health are in their infancy, but even so, they have opened a window on elder-pet health care that has far-reaching applications. Sometimes their influence reaches across species lines, and offers help and hope to aging humans. This exchange of information works in both directions, with human geriatric information also helping our dogs lead longer, healthier lives.

Golden Moments: Care from the Heart

Madelene Rutz of Eureka, Missouri, has loved dogs for as long as she can remember. Brook, though, is one of a kind. They've been together since the nine-year-old Doberman was a twelve-week-old puppy, and have always been extremely close. Through the years, the pair has competed together in a number of doggy sports, from obedience, tracking, and agility, to conformation. "I listen to my dogs," says Madelene, and she pays attention to what they tell her.

When Brook started limping last year, Madelene knew there was a problem.

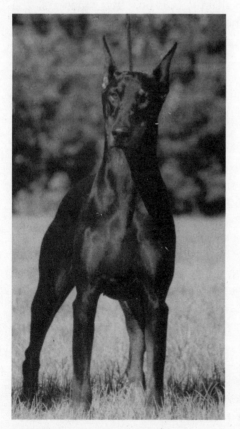

Brook's knee injury was repaired with surgery, and had her feeling like an energetic pup again. *(Photo Credit: Madelene Rutz)*

She took the dog to see Chesterfield-area veterinarian Dr. Ken Thornbery for an exam. "I rely heavily on Dr. Thornbery for my dogs, and have a tremendous amount of faith in him," says Madelene. He recommended first resting the leg to see if that would help. "That didn't seem to give any kind of results," says Madelene, "so Dr. Thornbery took X rays and sent them to the university for them to take a look."

Once they'd examined the X rays, the specialists also took a look at Brook. They diagnosed a ruptured anterior cruciate ligament (ACL). This is a common problem in both human and canine athletes. The ACL helps hold the knee together, and the injury causes a painful instability that can cripple the dog. Without repair, Brook would continue to limp, and the pain would eventually worsen and predispose her to arthritis.

Madelene scheduled surgery to repair the problem. She was told to keep the dog from exerting herself until the surgery.

Before the knee could be repaired, though, Brook turned the wrong way and really hurt herself. "She cried, and Brook is not a dog that shows pain. It hurt me, too, because there was nothing I could do," says Madelene. She called the university and explained that Brook was now in a terrific amount of pain, and asked if they could move up the date of the surgery. There were already a number of dogs in line ahead of Brook, though, and also in the same painful situation. "They put me on a waiting list."

Luckily Brook didn't have to wait long. Madelene got a phone call at work on April 13 that there had been a cancellation—could she get the dog to the university that same afternoon? "It's an hour-and-a-half drive to Columbia. And I was thinking, Oh, man, it's Friday the thirteenth!"

After some frantic last-minute arrangements to get off of work, Madelene managed to get Brook to the hospital in time for the surgery. "I had to say good-bye to her, give her a hug and kiss, and tell her I'd be back for her," says Madelene. "It's really hard leaving them when you're that far away."

Brook's ACL repair involved an innovative procedure called a tibial plateau leveling osteotomy, or TPLO. Rather than replacing the ruptured ligament, or attempting to stitch it back together, TPLO redesigns the bones that come together to form the knee. The surgeon, Dr. Jimmy Cook, cut the end of the tibia and rotated it so the flat part stayed level. That kept the femur from sliding off when the dog moved. This configuration no longer needs the anterior cruciate ligament to hold it together.

Madelene picked Brook up on Sunday and was sent home with pain medicine to give the dog over the next three days. Brook was restricted to light activity for six weeks after the surgery. She healed quickly and well, and since then has only rarely needed a buffered aspirin if she acts like her leg bothers her.

Brook is now back to normal and hasn't slowed down at all. "You'd never know she was nine," says Madelene, who never thought twice about getting help for her canine friend. Madelene loves all her dogs but says Brook is special. "She's my heart," says Madelene.

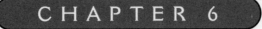

CHAPTER 6

Making Choices

In most cases, dogs will not outlive their owners. That's a sad fact every dog owner must face. But although they may live shorter lives, dogs seem to have a unique ability to pack many decades' worth of joy into their short time on this planet.

As responsible pet owners, we all face the knowledge that our dogs *may* develop an illness or infirmity. We understand that someday we *will* lose them to death. That in no way diminishes our love for them. In fact, it makes the time we share with our dogs even more cherished.

The longer they are with us, the more difficult those life and death decisions become. Should you prolong her life, or is that selfish? How do you know when the time is right? Cost of care, concerns over her comfort, and guilt about making these choices can make your time together even more difficult.

Please give yourself permission to stop, take a deep breath, and look at your dog. Know that she trusts you to make these decisions for her. She's not worried, and she won't "blame" you for making one choice over another. There is no wrong answer. All you can expect of yourself is to make informed choices with the best information you have. It doesn't matter what anybody else would choose—this is between you and your pet. *Any decision you make based on love and concern for her welfare cannot be wrong.*

THE FINAL GIFT

Dogs are born; dogs live; dogs die. Some die in tragic accidents, while others simply slip away in quiet old age. Others linger on and on, in continuous illness and decline. All deserve our love, but these last may rate our greatest gift of all—granting them a calm, gentle death through euthanasia.

When do you know the time has come?

"It's all the things you've heard," says Susan Wynn, DVM. "When they stop eating, when they stop enjoying being with you." When you begin to wonder, ask yourself this important question: how many more days will you get that are better than *today?* "I think that's one of the most meaningful measures," says Dr. Wynn. "If today is really bad, and almost every day following this is going to be as bad, it helps for you to make that call."

When injury or disease holds your dog in ongoing distress with little hope of recovery; when your dog gives up and longs for release; when a longer life is not a better life; these measures are ones only you, as your

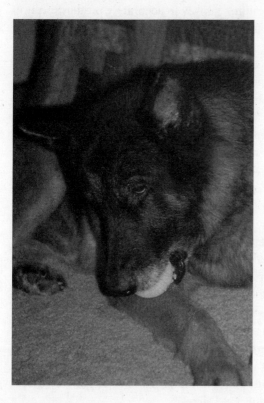

Fafnir loved his ball. He played with it, slept with it, and couldn't eat unless it was in his bowl so he could eat around it. Fafnir's ball games were a barometer of his health during his golden years. Changes in your dog's habits offer cues to help you judge his quality of life. *(Photo Credit: Amy D. Shojai)*

dog's best friend, can make. People who are very close to their dogs intuitively *know* when the time is right. Your dog will tell you when she's ready to say good-bye.

Preparing for the End

The best time to talk about pet loss is before you lose your dog. "The diagnosis of a terminal disease is often the time that the grieving process starts," says Laura Garret, DVM. "As veterinarians, we talk to clients about their thoughts and feelings. That's an important part of our job."

It's not unusual during the course of chronic treatment for owners to start to ask, What's going to happen in the end? What should I look for? This is a good thing, says Dr. Garret, because it helps eliminate surprises and prepares you for what to expect.

At the time of diagnosis, the veterinarian typically explains treatment options and prognosis. "If it's a cancer, I'll explain that we can prolong the life very comfortably but not cure them, and in the end, you will lose her to this disease," says Dr. Garret. There's no way to accurately predict survival, but the veterinarian can tell you the average survival time for the condition with a given treatment.

"For me, grief counseling is part of the therapeutic process," says Barbara Kitchell, DVM. As an oncologist, she treats primarily patients with metastatic cancer. "We know what the outcome is going to be; it's just a question of how long it takes to get there," she says. Treatment can cure some patients, she says, "but for the most part, cancer is tougher than we are, or smarter or more resilient. It's got time on its side. Cancer therapy *gives* time," she says. "You give time back that they wouldn't otherwise have." Treatment for any chronic disease also offers the owner time to come to grips with the reality of eventual loss.

In certain circumstances, owners may wish to take control in a situation that's otherwise out of their hands, and have the dog euthanized while she's still feeling good. Conditions like tumors, for example, may cause sudden seizures or hemorrhage, which may result in a traumatic, scary, and painful death. "They cannot stand the thought of coming home and finding their pet dead, or having the kids see this," says Dr. Garret. They don't want to have to rush her to the emergency room at two o'clock in the morning, where they may not know the vet on call, or have her die on the way to the clinic. "That's a horrible memory, with no beauty to it at all. They'd rather talk it over with the family, and plan a euthanasia, have the family there, have her favorite toys there," says Dr. Garret.

Other owners can't do that when the dog still looks and feels good. "I respect that, too," says Dr. Garret. "When she's fighting a terminal illness, any time really is the right time to decide to put her to sleep. It may help the process by giving you some control over it."

Talking to Children

The passing of a pet is often a child's first experience with death and loss of a loved one. It is important to make children a part of the process, and let them be involved, says Dr. Kitchell. She believes children can learn valuable lessons from the death of a pet, and that parents shouldn't fear involving them in the reality of the situation. Death is a painful but natural—and essential—part of life.

Being present during the euthanasia can be a gift to both the adults and children in the dog's life. Such passages into death are painless, calm, and loving. "This is not just about the biology," says Dr. Kitchell. "The relationship has to be honored and has to be respected. This is about the spiritual side of that bond between a person and an animal."

Children are directly affected by the way parents react. "They're the role models," says Wallace Sife, Ph.D., a psychologist specializing in pet bereavement. We must try to explain that all things must die, that even though pets live shorter lives, we become better people because of the wonderful love we share with them. "When they see the parent afraid of death, they're going to be frightened, too," says Dr. Sife. Often the younger the child, the easier it will be for them to accept that death is a normal process, and that the dog will go to doggy heaven.

In trying to help cushion the pain for a child, parents may lie about the situation, fudge the truth, or use euphemisms that in reality terrify the child. "Parents will say, 'God wanted him so much that he had to take him.' And the child then wonders, 'What about me? Doesn't God love me?'" says Dr. Sife. He cautions against using terms like *put to sleep*. He has counseled children who were terrified because of confusion over this phrase. Instead, he says we need to talk about the pet in a whole new way, in which his memory lives on in our hearts to make us better people.

Older children take less at face value. When the child is old enough to really comprehend, Dr. Sife recommends parents bring the child into the decision-making process. "The parent is going to decide," he says, "but let the child feel they're a part of it." This loving decision should be made as a group, rather than by individuals—the adults—who announce what will happen without consulting the children.

Teenagers especially should be involved in the discussion, and very often will oppose any decision made by their parents. Still, they need to be a part of a loving good-bye, and given the chance to understand how the process works. Should your teenagers strenuously object, delay the decision for a few days until they get used to the idea. When mutual love drives the decision, there's no conflict, says Dr. Sife. "The feeling of working together and memorializing the beloved pet can even help unify families that are having problems," he adds.

Right Time, Right Place

You have choices when it comes to ending your dog's life. Do you want to be present for the euthanasia? "I greatly prefer that, personally," says Dr. Garret. "Having owners there is a culmination of the pet's life. Most clients do choose to be there, and are happy, because it's a very peaceful process. They feel like they were with them to the last minute." Other owners want to remember their dog running around and happy, and prefer not to be present.

Veterinarians should respect your wishes, whatever they are, says Dr. Wynn. "You have to be offered that choice," she says. "If you're told you cannot be with your animal, run. This is something that most veterinarians now realize is part of the deal." Dr. Garret agrees. "It's very important to feel in the end that you had the sort of good-bye that you wanted," she says.

Some veterinarians will euthanize an animal at the owner's home, and feel that may be more comforting to the dog. You may choose to have an outdoor euthanasia if the weather is nice. "We'll take blankets outside, sit under a tree so it's not such a clinical environment," says Dr. Garret.

Other owners don't want to be reminded each time they walk into the room that Fluffy died there. "For some people that's a good feeling and for others it's not good," says Bill Fortney, DVM.

A home euthanasia allows the other pets in the family to say good-bye. It sometimes helps them to see the body after the animal has passed away, so they understand she's gone and they don't spend days or weeks searching and crying for their lost buddy. If you prefer to bring the dog into the clinic for euthanasia and are worried about other pets grieving, ask if you can bring them along, suggests Dr. Garret. However, she recommends that you wait until after euthanasia to bring in other pets, so that your whole focus can remain on the pet to whom you're saying good-bye.

Another option is to take the body home and allow the other cats and dogs to investigate. Be prepared for *any* reaction from the other pets. Some animals become extremely upset and howl and cry, while others don't even sniff the body. "No reaction may make owners feel worse, and think he doesn't even care," says Dr. Garret. That's not really true, she says; it's just the way that animal deals with death. After life has fled, he may recognize it's not the same dog anymore.

Most commonly, euthanasia takes place in the veterinarian's office. When your veterinarian has provided long-term care for your dog, it is a sad day for the vet as well. Euthanasia is a culmination of everyone's relationship together in helping an animal to die comfortably and peacefully, with all the loved ones around her, including the veterinarian. "There are times we cry with the owner during the procedure. You can cry because you feel bad for the owners and you're saying good-bye to the pet yourself," says Dr. Garret. "The time when I can go through euthanasia without feeling any emotion is the time I'll quit. I don't want to get to that point."

Understanding Euthanasia

Today, many clinics provide a separate room that allows you to have private time alone with your dog before, during, and after the euthanasia. The first step typically involves placing a catheter in the vein, to make it easier to administer the euthanasia solution when the time comes. Chronically ill dogs may already have an IV catheter in place.

Dr. Garret prefers to place the catheter in the back leg. A rear-leg placement allows the owner to interact with the dog's face throughout the procedure. "We'll actually use a butterfly catheter, which is a long extension, so we're not right up by the leg," she explains. "We can be a little way away with the syringes and not be crowding the animal." Occasionally the dog will be sedated first, which makes her very sleepy. You may prefer to forgo the sedation, so that she remains alert up to the end, and you are better able to interact with the dog you know and love during your good-byes.

Once you have had time to visit, the veterinarian will return and ask if you're ready. The procedure should be explained to you in advance, so you know what to expect. As the drug relaxes the dog, sometimes she will involuntarily urinate, so if you want to hold your dog you may want to cuddle her in a towel. If the dog has not been sedated before, she may receive that injection now so she's relaxed and has a smoother transition. Then a slow IV injection of the euthanasia solution, a barbiturate anesthetic-type drug, is administered. It can be very quick-acting; usually within a minute or two the dog will be gone. The veterinarian will listen for a heartbeat to confirm that the dog is dead.

"After the pet is gone and the heartbeat stops, sometimes they will twitch or have last-minute breaths. But it's not them," says Dr. Garret. "They're gone at that point; it's just an automatic response by the body." At this point, most people wish to spend some time alone with their pet. Don't hesitate to ask for this consideration if it's not offered.

The way euthanasia is handled will color the way you feel about your veterinarian in the future. "Several studies show that about 60 percent of owners who have their animal put to sleep will change veterinarians," says Dr. Fortney. There are a variety of reasons for this. Perhaps the most telling is that no matter how wonderful the veterinarian may have been, some folks just don't like going back to the practice where they put Fluffy to sleep.

VALIDATING GRIEF

Elizabeth Kübler-Ross is known for her work documenting the five stages of grief people feel at the loss of a human loved one. The stages are denial, anger, bargaining, (*I'll do X, Y, Z, if only he'll be okay*), depression, and finally acceptance. You will feel these same emotions to varying degrees after the loss of a beloved pet. Grieving is a normal human process.

A major loss of any kind will produce a sense of bereavement, but pet bereavement has unique qualities because we share very different parts of our lives with pets. "We have to understand specifically what the bond was, why it is so valid to grieve this way, and not belittle ourselves or doubt ourselves," says Dr. Sife. We look on our pets as dependent children. Even more, an old pet may represent milestones in your own life—the dog was a childhood chum, accompanied you to college, and was there for your wedding. Losing her feels like losing a part of yourself.

Pet bereavement is also more difficult to navigate because you may not receive the same sympathy and support that you would if you'd lost a human family member. "Many people almost resent the fact that we can bereave so deeply for a pet," says Dr. Sife. "They will take it personally and get very judgmental or offensive." Part of that reaction stems from society's negative view of death, which makes it difficult to openly express grief, especially for "only" a pet. "For that reason throughout history people have pretty much stayed in the closet with their grief when a pet dies," says Dr. Sife.

People who have never experienced a close relationship with a pet have the most difficult time understanding our pain. That can be especially hard to deal with in families where perhaps one member was much closer to the dog than others. "I feel really sorry for people who don't have that capacity to understand the bond," says Dr. Kitchell. "It's as if they go through life color-blind. There's a dimension of life they can't appreciate."

Each person experiences grief in different ways. The process can be short or long, and the stages of grief are not necessarily sequential—you may feel depression, then denial and anger, for example. "You do not have to experience all these stages to successfully grieve," says Dr. Garret. While the dog's illness may throw you into deep denial, your husband may simply get angry—or come to terms with the dog's death much more quickly than you are able.

Guilt is common, even when you made all the *right* choices with your veterinarian's help. The *would have, should have, could haves* will only cause you to lose sleep and prolong the pain. Have faith in yourself that you made the best decisions for your dog at that moment in time. Your dog couldn't have a better testimony to your love.

Sometimes there may be a delay of grief. At first you feel no emotion—again, there is no right or wrong to the process. Delayed grief may come days, weeks, even months later, when the sight of Fluffy's Christmas stocking with embroidered bones on the front causes an emotional meltdown.

All of these faces of grief are normal.

"The important factor here is that someone is hurting. And if we are good humans, whether we agree or disagree with the reasons, we give compassion," says Dr. Sife.

Even very close family members and friends who are very loving and want to help may not know how to support you. They'll say, "Don't cry." Or they'll try to diminish the reason for the pain by saying, "It's only a dog." "That, of course, only intensifies the pain and causes alienation and distancing, and can even damage or permanently destroy friendships," says Dr. Sife.

What is the *right* thing to say to help a friend, comfort a family member, or guide your children through their grief? If you loved the pet, or are a pet owner yourself, you can commiserate from firsthand experience and knowledge. If you're not a pet owner, and you care for the person, simply ask how you can help. Acknowledge that they're going through something terrible that you don't really understand and haven't experienced. Then tell them you care for them and want to be there for them.

Often just a supportive, nonjudgmental presence is the most important salve in the healing process. Listen to their cherished stories about the special dog—the way she always stole the covers each morning to wake them, how she'd catch Frisbees for hours on end, the way she always met them at the door.

When you are the person grieving, remember that you are not alone. Every person reading this book loves or has loved a dog, and understands the pain of losing a beloved canine friend. You may feel numb, an aching emptiness that something special is now missing. It may catch you by surprise when entering a room—and she's not there racing to greet you. Her food bowls are still on the kitchen floor, with the last bit of water or kibble she left behind. You stub a toe on that darn rawhide chew, and dissolve in tears, knowing this time when you put it away she won't drag it back into the clutter. Maybe you "feel" her leap onto the bed at night as you doze off to sleep, or "see" her out of the corner of your eye. These are all normal experiences, and common to people who have shared a particularly close bond with their dog.

It's normal to feel awful. It hurts terribly, but you are not crazy. Aren't other things such as work or people supposed to be more important? No. Your pet and grief are no less important, just important in a different way. She had a unique impact on your life, or you wouldn't miss her the way you do.

Please always remember that there is no guilt or shame in being a caring person. Do not let anyone make you feel wrong for honoring your pet with tears.

The first line of defense is support from people who've been through it themselves. Talk about your feelings. Remember her by sharing stories with other pet lovers. Local veterinarians or animal shelters may offer grief-support groups that meet in your area. There are also pet-loss support hot lines from a number of veterinary universities. If you are on the Internet, a number of pet sites provide pet-loss support groups where you can share stories, cry a little, receive—and give—support to other pet lovers going down the same emotional path.

"The grief process can be abnormally long, and people can get sort of *stuck* at one stage or another," says Dr. Garret. "In some cases, it's a very good idea to see a health care professional." Dr. Sife says the loss of a pet may sometimes trigger other very deep-rooted and unresolved problems in the person's life that they may not even recognize, or have repressed. "Then they're overwhelmed with grief and they can only see it as the loss of the pet, which is intense by itself," he says. "That's where it takes a professional counselor who is professionally trained and capable of identifying and helping the person."

COMFORT ZONE

Memorializing your dog can be a comfort to you and a tribute to his life. Memorials can be expensive purchases, such as a grave marker, or something as simple as creating a scrapbook of memories. There is no right or wrong way to memorialize your dog, and creative remembrances that are individual to you will mean the most.

- Write a letter or poem to your dog. Tributes can be posted at www.in-memory-of-pets.org/tributes.asp or other sites. She can even be honored in a "virtual" pet cemetery, such as www.rainbowsbridge.com, and www.mycemetery.com.
- Donate money in your pet's honor to a worthy animal organization.
- Commission a portrait from an animal artist.
- Inscribe a headstone, grave marker, or other keepsake with your dog's name. Garden Grace (877-252-1221, www.gardenstones.net) offers pet memorial slate stepping stones, and Reflections In Time (252-514-4494, www.reflectionsintime.net) custom-engraves slate and glassware for pet memorials and wall plaques.
- Make a pawprint impression. World by the Tail (970-223-5753) sells a kit for about $10 with molding clay that's baked in the oven. Pawprints (800-827-6985, www.pearhead.com) also offers a kit.
- Choose an urn or container for cremation remains. Pro Connection (877-4-OUR PET, www.proconxn.com) uses fossil stones with inside storage for the pet's tag, lock of fur, toy, or cremated ashes. GoodWorks (888-586-8400, www.4goodworks.com) custom-designs porcelain urns and decorates them with a photo of your pet. BrandNew Memorial Markers (800-964-8251, www.brandnewpetmarkers.com) are hardwood urns with a custom copper plaque with the pet's personal information.

HONORING THE MEMORY

Remembering your dog can be a helpful part of grieving. Part of that includes the decision of what becomes of her body. When the pet has been a patient at a teaching hospital at a university, the veterinarian may ask you to consider granting permission for an autopsy, especially if it's an unusual case. "It may help other pets," says Dr. Garret. Some owners consider this a legacy that will live on and positively impact the lives of other dogs.

Ask your veterinarian for suggestions on how to handle her body. Some practices contract with services that take care of this for clients, particularly when the owner does not have the ability or resources to make other arrangements.

When you live in a rural area and have property available, a home burial may be your preference. Some cities have laws prohibiting the burial of pets within residential areas, so check with officials in your area. A home interment allows you to create a memorial grave site in a setting familiar to the missing canine friend—perhaps beneath a favorite tree she loved.

Pet cemeteries are now available in many locations and offer a "formal" burial arrangement that may include the plot, the casket, a gravestone or marker with inscription, or even a burial service. Pet cemeteries can be expensive. Ask your vet for a referral or check the yellow pages for local listings.

Cremation has become a popular choice, particularly for urban pet owners. It's typically less expensive than a cemetery. The pet's ashes can be kept in a container of your choice in your home or garden, or even scattered in a memorial ceremony. Ask your vet for local referral.

Many pet owners have funeral ceremonies, or memorials such as planting a tree or making a charitable donation in memory of a beloved pet. There is no wrong choice. "We make an impression of the paw," says Dr. Garret. "A lot of times owners like to take a lock of fur with a ribbon around it," she says. "Little things like that really help an owner through the grieving process."

Some formalized type of memorial can be particularly helpful to children, says Dr. Sife. "We have to show children that bereavement is a loving process of remembrance."

After the death of a dog, some people will never be ready for another pet. Others are ready immediately. No two people are going to react the same way. Very often, after a time, owners celebrate their dog's life not by replacing her, but by remembering her with another of her kind. It's not uncommon for owners to say that the deceased pet "sent" the new one. After all, other dogs need you, and such unselfish love should not be wasted.

Death is a natural process. It will come despite our best efforts to delay the inevitable. But it does not have to be scary or painful—dying can, in fact, be a beautiful, loving experience for both you and your dog. "We are the best memorials that we can create for our pets," says Dr. Sife. "If we can make our lives better because of them, that is a wonderful tribute."

PART TWO

A-to-Z Health Concerns

Arthritis

Arthritis is a degenerative disease of the joints. Inflammation and degradation of the cartilage in the joints cause progressively worsening pain and disability as the dog ages.

Cartilage covers the end of the bones that come together to form joints. This specialized tissue cushions the contact and allows the bones to move freely against each other. A joint capsule encases the entire joint, and contains a membrane that produces a lubricating fluid that maintains cartilage health. The natural motion of the joint pumps this synovial fluid where it's needed.

Damage and inflammation develop when misaligned or malformed bones fit imperfectly in the joint and cause erosion of the cartilage when it rubs together. Loose or torn tendons, which normally hold the bones in place, cause joint instability that leads to arthritis. Injury to the cartilage from trauma, such as broken bones, also predisposes the dog to arthritis as he ages. In addition, injured cartilage releases inflammation-causing enzymes, which interfere with elasticity, and the ability of the joint capsule to nourish and repair itself. The resulting pain causes dogs to restrict movement, which further reduces the distribution of the synovial fluid and causes more damage.

Large-breed dogs have a greater incidence of arthritis because their greater weight places more stress on the joints. Certain breeds may be more likely to develop arthritis because of inherited tendencies. "Labradors are little lemons as far as orthopedics," says Dr. Kathleen Linn.

"Bernese Mountain Dogs in this country are kind of orthopedic disasters." She says Rottweilers and Labradors are prone to knee problems, while Boxers and German Shepherds are moderately prone. Any dog can develop arthritis, though, and they become more susceptible the older they get.

SENIOR SYMPTOMS

"Dogs almost never cry out when they're in pain from sore joints," says Kathleen Linn, DVM, an orthopedic surgeon at the University of Wisconsin. "Owners frequently don't think their animals are in pain until they're having a really tough time getting around." Arthritis is progressive. It becomes worse as time goes on. The most typical signs are changes in the dog's activity:

- Reluctance to go on long walks is the most common sign. "They tire easily when they are on a walk, and can't exercise as much as they used to," says Dr. Mike Conzemius.
- Circling endlessly before lying down or struggling to get up are also very common.
- Mornings are usually worse. Movement warms up the joints, and mobility often improves later in the day.
- There will be more of a reluctance to jump up onto or off of the couch or the bed, or into or out of the car or truck.
- Avoiding stairs is typical. Reluctance to go up or down stairs or jump up or down are the principle signs of arthritis in multiple joints.
- Limping or holding up a paw or leg may point to a single joint or leg that's affected, says Dr. Linn. When the same joints on both sides (i.e., both hips) are affected, dogs tend to mask discomfort more easily.

The most common joints affected are the hips, elbows, and knees. Dr. Linn says hip and elbow arthritis almost always develop as a consequence of dysplasia in the joint. "Dysplasia is a developmental disease they start having as puppies," she says. Although dysplasia may show up as pain when the animal is a year or two old, oftentimes the dog is able to compensate and owners won't notice any problem. "Then it starts catching up with them at around six or seven years of age," says Linn. One of the most common causes of lameness—that is, limping or holding up a leg—is knee arthritis. "That is almost always secondary to a torn cruciate ligament," says Linn.

Arthritis is usually diagnosed based on symptoms and X rays. Sometimes a force-plate test helps determine how much weight the dog is placing on each leg. The dog is led across a platform (force plate) that's connected to a computer, which measures function. Force-plate tests are also used to measure improvement after therapy is begun. Once arthritis is diagnosed, therapy consists of any one or a combination of surgery, physical therapy, medical management (drugs), weight control, and acupuncture.

AGE-DEFYING TIPS

Arthritis almost always develops as a result of joint injury earlier in life, so prompt repair or treatment prevents problems later. "There are surgeries that can be done at a young age for elbow or hip dysplasia which are effective," says Dr. Linn. However, these surgeries are effective only when performed before arthritic changes occur.

Once your old dog has any degree of arthritis, you can slow the progression and even reverse some of the signs, says Dr. Conzemius.

- Keep dogs active. Low-impact exercise such as walking or swimming is ideal to help keep joints from stiffening.
- Keep dogs thin. Added weight puts more stress upon joints. Regular exercise along with a reduced-calorie "senior" diet helps reduce or control weight.

NONSURGICAL TREATMENT

"Our goals are to decrease pain, increase function, and increase quality of life and slow down progression," says James L. Cook, DVM. Defining goals is important, particularly when dealing with aged arthritic pets. A cure is not possible—once the damage is done, arthritis won't get better, although the severity of the symptoms can be reduced.

Not only must owners decide on goals and define success, they must also monitor treatment to measure success. "We give them this report card they fill out so we can tell if the whole program is working," says Dr. Cook. The client must actively participate in the treatment in order to achieve and identify success, he says. Modifications to the treatment plan can be made once you know how it is working.

Nonsurgical management of arthritis follows a three-part approach. It incorporates weight control, exercise, and pain relief using medication, acupuncture, or other therapies.

Weight Control

"The dogs that have the worst problems with arthritis are ones that are overweight," says Dr. Linn. "Slimming them down is probably the single most important thing we do."

If anything, dogs should be on the thin side and look underweight, says Dr. Cook. "You almost want your neighbors to say, 'I wonder if they're feeding their dog?'!" On the Purina Body Condition Score he recommends the dog fall around a 4 or 5 on that scale. "You should be able to feel the ribs and see the waist," he says.

Exercise

The second step is moderate exercise. "It's better for them to get up and move around than to just lie around the house all day," says Dr. Linn. "The best exercise, the most perfect, is swimming. It gets all the joints to go through a good range of motion without weight bearing." Swimming is also good for the cardiovascular system.

When you don't have access to a pool, or your dog dislikes water, walks are a great alternative. "Slow walks on a leash are fairly low impact, it doesn't bang on the joints like a dog that's bouncing around the backyard after squirrels," says Dr. Linn.

Ten minutes a couple times a day is a good start, says Dr. Conzemius. Small amounts of daily exercise are much better than marathon sessions once a week. Massage before and after exercise can help keep muscles from tightening, which can make your dog reluctant to get off his furry tail. Massage also doubles as a nice bonding exercise.

Medication

There are advantages and disadvantages to each arthritis medication, says Dr. Cook. What works best in your dog may not be helpful in another—but often you won't know until you try. Generally he recommends a three-week trial on any medication. The results are monitored, and if it's not working, another drug can be tried.

"Sometimes I'll just start with buffered aspirin or Ascriptin because it's cheap, over-the-counter, and it works in a lot of dogs," he says. Ascriptin is aspirin coated with Maalox to help prevent gastric irritation. "Most dogs tolerate aspirin well. The big side effect of aspirin is stomach ulcers," says

Dr. Linn. "That manifests itself as a lack of appetite, vomiting, or dark stools." Other human medicines, such as Tylenol, ibuprofen, and naproxin sodium, are not recommended.

FEEDING FOR HEALTH

Reduced-calorie diets are helpful to slim down an overweight dog and help take the strain off arthritic joints. Regular "senior" formulas may do the trick, but in some cases a veterinary-supervised diet is required. Some foods also contain ingredients designed to help ease the discomfort of achy joints. Some options include:

- Nutro Natural Choice Senior
- Waltham Canine Mobility Support Diet
- Eukanuba Veterinary Diets, Nutritional Weight Maintenance Formula, Senior Plus/Canine
- Eukanuba Veterinary Diets, Nutritional Weight Loss Formulas Restricted-Calorie/Canine
- Hill's Prescription Diet Canine r/d (reduction diet)
- Hill's Prescription Diet Canine w/d (weight diet)
- IVD Select Care Canine Hifactor Formula
- IVD Select Care Canine Mature Formula
- IVD Select Care Canine Vegetarian Formula
- Nutro Max Weight Control Formula
- Precise Light Formula for Less Active or Overweight Dogs
- Purina Veterinary Diets, OM Overweight Management Formula
- Waltham Canine Calorie Control Diet

NSAIDs—nonsteroidal anti-inflammatory drugs—are a class of medication that can be very helpful to arthritic dogs. They work by affecting the production of certain enzymes that are involved in joint inflammation and pain, says Dr. Linn. Carprofen, trade name Rimadyl, works in a great many dogs. "The very rare dog does have liver problems with it," she says. "I recommend checking for liver problems [through a blood test] prior to administering it, watching how they react to it, and rechecking blood a month after you first start it, and then after three months." Rimadyl is a pill given twice a day.

Another drug called etodolac, brand name Etogesic, works in a similar way to Rimadyl, but some owners consider it more convenient since it's given only once a day. "It's a little less likely to cause liver problems in dogs," says Dr. Linn. "It can cause stomach upset, but it's a little less likely to do that than aspirin." Dogs who have elevated liver enzymes and don't tolerate aspirin well could benefit from Etogesic.

Other drugs may be used less frequently because of potential side effects. Ketoprofen is a good analgesic but has more of a tendency to cause stomach ulcers than does Rimadyl. Peroxicam is another NSAID, also used to treat certain cancers. "It is an excellent pain reliever, but it's not the one we usually reach for first because it has a greater tendency to cause ulcers," says Dr. Linn.

"Most NSAIDs block both the COX-I and COX-II pathways," says Dr. Conzemius. These pathways are the specific biochemical mechanisms the drug acts upon to cause pain relief. But blocking the COX-I pathway causes complications that affect kidney function, stomach erosions, and ulcers, he says. "COX-II pathway is mostly for inflammatory mediators so [blocking that pathway] reduces swelling and painful joints."

A medication that's specific only to the COX-II is ideal for treating arthritis. Currently there is no COX-II inhibitor drug approved specifically for use in dogs, but human drugs can be very safe and effective if used correctly. Human products available include Celebrex and Vioxx. "We use these off-label, just like we do with all of our antibiotics, for example," says Dr. Conzemius.

Nutraceuticals

Today, a variety of nutritional supplements—nutraceuticals—are used like drugs to treat a wide range of health conditions. Also called "functional foods," these are substances intended to maintain or improve health beyond what ordinary nutrients in the food provide. Subclassifications include herbs and other plant materials, enzymes, animal extracts, and other chemical compounds or microbial products. For example, the beneficial bacteria in acidophilus—plain yogurt you buy from the supermarket—will help rebalance the normal population of bacteria in the dog's intestines and allow dogs to better absorb their food.

Some of the newest "senior" diets for dogs contain nutraceuticals that are said to benefit joint health, and are helpful for arthritic pets. It's also possible to add appropriate supplements to your dog's diet. For example, Dr. Linn says essential fatty acids, specifically the omega-3 fatty acids, can help with arthritis pain. "A lot of folks prescribe a combination supplement called DermCaps," she says. Holistic veterinarians may recommend herbal supplements, such as *Boswellia serrata,* which is said to naturally fight joint inflammation, and is commonly used by people in India. Products that contain green-lipped mussels (perna mussel), such as Glyco-Flex, are helpful because they contain GAG-like compounds (glycosaminoglycan), which have been shown to slow the degeneration of cartilage in the joints. Perna mussels also smell fishy, which dogs really like.

GAG and proteoglycan compounds help slow the progression of arthritis by protecting the joint cartilage, says Dr. Cook. "We've actually done some of the research here, and other labs have verified it, that these nutraceuticals, especially the glucosamines, work as an antidegradative," says Dr. Cook. He particularly likes using these products because they have no side effects and can be used along with other medications.

Compounds such as chondroitin and glucosamine also have anti-inflammatory properties, says Dr. Conzemius. "They can reduce swelling, and that can help with the pain." These supplements are probably most effective in dogs that have only mild arthritis. He says they don't "prevent" arthritis but they may modulate or slow the progression and therefore may be helpful in dogs who have not yet developed symptoms but are at risk for the disease.

Some compounds work better than others, says Dr. Cook. The chondroitin sulfates are fine, he says, but are probably broken down further in the gut, so you skip a step by giving glucosamine products from the beginning. "The glucosamine HCL is probably the best," he says, because it's better absorbed into the joint. "I just have people buy the glucosamine HCL over the counter."

The nutraceutical industry is not well regulated. The effectiveness and quality of products varies greatly from brand to brand, and claims made on some labels have been found to be false. A glucosamine and chondroitin sulfate combination product, called Cosequin, is one of the few that's actually been tested in scientific trials, and it is most often recommended by veterinarians. It is, however, more expensive than many health food products.

Dr. Cook suggests looking on the label specifically for the 500-milligram dosage of glucosamine HCL. He recommends that dogs under fifty pounds receive 500 milligrams once a day; fifty- to eighty-pound dogs 500 milligrams twice a day; and dogs over eighty pounds should get a total of 1,500 milligrams, usually two 500-milligram capsules in the morning and one in the evening. "The most I'd do would be a thousand milligrams twice a day for the real big dog," says Dr. Cook. "But once we're getting a good effect, then we try and figure out the minimal dose that's effective, and back them off over time."

About ten years go, an injectable drug called polysulfated glycosaminoglycan (PSGAG) was commonly used in horses for cartilage injuries. Today,

Adequan has been FDA-approved as a disease-modifying osteoarthritis drug for dogs. It is similar to the oral glucosamine-type drugs, but when given by injection, the concentrated dose can have a more dramatic effect. It doesn't work for all patients, warns Dr. Linn. "Fifty to 60 percent of the patients I've treated with Adequan show response from a little better to 'Hallelujah! I can walk!' For the ones it doesn't help, it is just expensive," she says. The latest recommendation suggests two milligrams per pound of body weight by intramuscular injection, twice weekly for up to eight injections. It generally takes two or three injections before you notice any change.

NURSE ALERT!

- A number of arthritis medications are available. Nearly all are in pill form, and will require you to pill your dog one or more times a day.
- Many dogs enjoy and benefit from massage, especially from someone they love.
- Following surgery, you may be required to keep incisions or bandages clean, restrict your dog's movement, or encourage him in physical therapy activities.

Acupuncture

Acupuncture falls into its own category—it is not a drug, but can act like one to relieve the pain of arthritis. It can be used along with other drug therapies. "It's not uncommon for me to have an animal that's on carprofen or Rimadyl, plus also getting some acupuncture and perhaps some of the nutraceuticals," says Bill Fortney, DVM. "I think that's very appropriate."

Dogs that are unable to tolerate a particular medicine due to liver problems or other concerns may benefit from the pain relief of acupuncture. "It certainly has no ill effects," says Dr. Linn. "It's very noninvasive; it's safe. That's certainly one that's worth a go."

SURGICAL TREATMENT

Some dogs do extremely well with nonsurgical management, so that's always the first thing to try, says Dr. Conzemius. "There's a significant emotional and financial investment owners make when they go for [surgery], so it makes perfect sense to try a little aspirin or nonsteroidal prior to jumping into joint replacement," he says.

COMFORT ZONE

- Ramps make it easier for the arthritic dog to reach the bed or sofa. Commercial ramps are available in different sizes. BedderBacks Dog Bed Ramps are available at www.bedderbacks.com.
- Offer elevated food bowls to minimize neck or back strain.
- Heated beds help ease the pain of achy, stiff joints. Products come with built-in electric heating pads. The Snuggle Safe plate-size pad (available from Drs. Foster & Smith) can be microwaved, then slipped beneath the dog's bed to warm without electricity.
- Fill a couple of socks with dry uncooked rice and microwave. They'll hold the heat and work great as doggy bed warmers.
- Wrap the dog in towels or blankets fresh from the dryer once a day for five minutes to warm up the muscles and relieve stiffness and pain.

But do consider surgery as a viable option. "So many people tell me they put their last dog to sleep because he had bad hips. Gee, that's the most curable disease we've got!" says Dr. Linn.

For many arthritic cases, the most effective treatment addresses the bad joint. "Knee surgery is the most effective way to treat a cruciate rupture and get a dog out of pain and back on his feet," says Dr. Linn. "Bad hips can certainly cripple but there are great surgeries that can give the dog back his old quality of life."

Over the past five to ten years, the likelihood of owners pursuing advanced treatments such as surgery has increased, says Dr. Conzemius. "There are more surgeons that can do these techniques, so it's more available to people. And owners are becoming better informed about what the disease is and the treatment options."

Here are a few of the most common—and some brand-new—surgical options for helping your aging dog deal with the pain of arthritis.

Total Hip Replacement

The best-known procedure, the Cadillac of joint repair, is total hip replacement, in which prosthetic joints replace the diseased arthritic ones. Dr. Linn says the surgery is 95 percent successful for athletic function in the hips, but it is pricey. The majority of dogs seem to do just fine with one total hip replacement and compensate fine. "The oldest dog I've done was fourteen," she says, "and most are six to ten years old. It's a big surgery, but most dogs walk on the hip they had surgery on, almost without lameness, the very day they go home." There is a recovery period in which the dog must be kept quiet and on a leash.

Femoral Head Ostectomy (FHO)

Most dogs with advanced arthritis in their hips have worn the cartilage right off the bones, so it's bone rubbing on bone. "It always looks to me like that highly polished marble in lobbies. You can imagine that hurts," says Dr. Linn. There's no cartilage left to protect. A better way to deal with the problem is to get rid of the bone-on-bone rubbing. The surgeon removes the ball part of the ball-and-socket joint in the hip, and closes the joint capsule over the socket. The dog forms a little pad of scar tissue and the hip joint is supported entirely by the muscles.

"It's a highly successful procedure, very good at getting animals out of pain," says Dr. Linn. The success rate is 80 to 85 percent, and FHO can be done even in big dogs. "I've done it on both hips in a bunch of Saint Bernards, for example, and once even in a camel," says Dr. Linn. Many veterinarians in general practice are very familiar with FHO, so it doesn't require going to a special center for orthopedics. It's less expensive than total hip replacement, but won't be as solid a joint, and most big dogs maintain a little bit of a Mae West butt wiggle. They tend to fatigue after very heavy exercise.

Total Elbow Replacement

For dogs with severe elbow arthritis, Dr. Conzemius and his colleagues have been working on developing a total elbow replacement procedure for about five years, and have performed the surgery for over two years. "We see all ages, but typically deal with large-breed dogs eight years old and older," he says. "We get good to excellent results in about 85 percent of our cases." The prosthetic joint is specific to veterinary medicine. It parallels knee replacement in people. "After total elbow replacement, aggressive physical therapy is essential," says Dr. Conzemius.

STEM CELL TECHNOLOGY

Large-breed dogs such as Golden Retrievers, Labrador Retrievers, Newfoundlands, Bernese Mountain Dogs, and Rottweilers are prone to elbow dysplasia, a painful disease that occurs when the joints don't line up properly and cartilage becomes damaged. Dr. P. R. Vulliet, Dr. Kurt Schulz, and colleagues at the School of Veterinary Medicine at the University of California—Davis believe that stem cells can enhance treatment for dogs suffering from elbow dysplasia.

Stem cells, developed and stored in the bone marrow, await further instruction from the body before they mature into a final form, such as cartilage. Stem cells can be gathered from the dog's body with very few side effects, and preliminary studies show stem cells injected into the damaged cartilage may prompt self-repair in as little as three to six months. Results of the one-year study, funded by Morris Animal Foundation, should be available in 2003.

Joint "Washout"

Arthroscopy employs a flexible tube with fiber optics that permits the veterinarian to see the inside of the joint through tiny noninvasive incisions. A procedure called "washout" has been shown to be very effective in people with arthritis, and is now being applied to arthritic dogs with the help of arthroscopy. Basically, the joint and tissue are debrided—scoured to remove damaged tissue and loose material—then washed clean. That not only gets rid of foreign matter; it also dilutes the biological chemicals that cause inflammation, says Dr. Cook. "We kind of slow down that process and make the joint feel better," he says. About 80 percent of people will have marked improvement for two to five years. "If you think about that in terms of an old dog, two to five years is pretty significant," he adds.

Tibial Plateau Leveling Osteotomy (TPLO)

Arthritis of the knee is almost always due to a ruptured cruciate ligament. Although a sudden tear can happen, more often the ligament frays and tears bit by bit, causing a progressive problem until the whole joint pops. This type of injury in large dogs rarely does well without surgery, says Dr. Linn. About 50 percent of small dogs do "okay" without surgery.

There are more than 40 different surgical repairs for this condition.

BOTTOM LINE

Cost for arthritis treatment varies depending on the specific product, procedure, and part of the country in which you live. For example:

- "For a Labrador-size dog, treatment with Cosequin in the bottle dose at our hospital is about $30 a month. But you can often kind of titrate back the dose once you've started them on that," says Dr. Linn.
- Hip replacement runs from $2000 to $4000 per side. "At our institution [University of Missouri] it's about $2500 to $2700 for a total hip replacement," says Dr. Cook.
- "Here [at University of Wisconsin] a femoral neck and head excision (FHO) runs about $1100 per side," says Dr. Linn.

Stitching the tear back together or attempting to replace the ligament may be helpful. Currently, a two-year study conducted by Dr. Paul Manley, of the University of Wisconsin—Madison, is evaluating the effectiveness of using a hamstring graft to repair the injury.

One of the most recent and successful procedures changes the dynamic of the knee joint. Dr. Cook first uses arthroscopy to see the injury. He cleans everything up and washes out the joint, and then performs a TPLO. The ends of the bone that come together to form the knee are restructured, so that one bone (the femur) can't slide off the other (the tibia) when the dog stands. After the surgery, the joint no longer needs a ligament for stability. "These dogs do almost too well," he says. "They're running out of here two days later wanting to stand on their back limbs and run and jump. Makes me nervous!"

Joint Fusion

In some instances, in a process called athrodesis, the painful joint can be eliminated entirely by fusing the two bones together, says Dr. Conzemius. Athrodesis can be performed in the knee, elbow, ankle, wrist, or hock. It leaves the dog with a limp due to lost mobility, but eliminates the pain of the joint. "With fusion of the hock, the wrist or ankle area, dogs do quite well," says Dr. Conzemius. "Mobility is more affected when they have arthrodesis of the knee or elbow."

Arthroscopic Joint Capsule Shrinkage

One of the newest treatments for joint instability employs thermal techniques to shrink the joint capsule. The research of Dr. Mark Markel, an orthopedic surgeon at the University of Wisconsin veterinary school, helped develop the procedure now used in human athletes called Electrothermal Assisted Capsulorphy, or ETAC. Today it is used in veterinary medicine to treat cruciate ligament injuries, hip dysplasia, and shoulder problems. "I just reported the first ten [shoulder] cases we did at the Veterinary Orthopedic Society meeting," says Dr. Cook. "All the dogs have really improved."

ARTHRITIS REPORT CARD
Patient:
Month:

Week 1

Attitude: Normal Depressed Agitated Comments:

Appetite: Normal Decreased Increased Comments:

Body Condition: 1 2 3 4 5 6 7 8 9 Weight (optional):
**Purina Body Condition System™—www.purina.com

Activity: Type Walking Running Playing
Duration
Frequency

Pain: At rest 0 1 2 3 4 5 6 7 8 9

Morning 0 1 2 3 4 5 6 7 8 9

Walking 0 1 2 3 4 5 6 7 8 9

Running/Playing 0 1 2 3 4 5 6 7 8 9
**visual analog scale: 0 = no pain to 9 = severe pain

Medications: Type medicine dose given days missed
name how
often

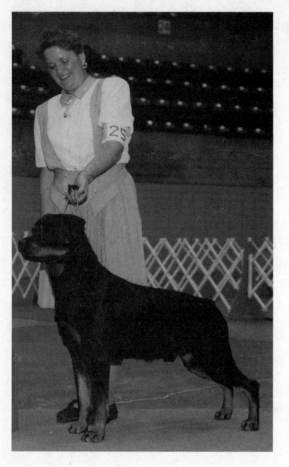

Hawk's innovative shoulder surgery put him back on his feet. *(Photo Credit: Melia Photography, courtesy of Kent Foster)*

Golden Moments: Smiles for Hawk

Double D Idaho Joe Hawk ("Hawk" for short) made history four years ago, when he was the first dog to undergo an experimental surgery on his shoulder. A limp affected Hawk's gait and interfered with his show career, says owner Kent Foster of Kent City, Missouri. "I think he injured it jumping out of the truck, but over time it got worse," says Kent.

Despite the discomfort, the beautiful Rottweiler's temperament was perfect. "He's very friendly to people and loves kids," says Kent. Hawk even smiles when he's happy—a mannerism Kent says he inherited from his father. The pain wasn't prompting any smiles, though, and Hawk's jumps had turned to limps.

Ken took Hawk to his veterinarian to figure out what was wrong. He was told the dog needed reconstructive surgery on his shoulder. "That would have put him out of commission for a long time, and it didn't sound like something I wanted to do," says Kent. "Hawk's my buddy. I wanted the best for him." He'd had a good experience with the veterinary school at University of Missouri in the past when Hawk's father had been treated, so Ken asked for a referral.

Veterinary orthopedic surgeon Dr. James Cook inserted an instrument called an arthroscope into the joint to examine the damage. The injured area was also injected with a specialized dye that made the tissue light up under the X-ray equipment, says Kent. That allowed them to see exactly what was wrong with Hawk's shoulder. "He had blown his shoulder out. It was torn up," says Kent. Without the repair, Hawk would most certainly develop arthritis that became even more painful as he got older.

Usually, surgery to repair such extensive shoulder damage requires a large incision, and a months-long rehabilitation period. Instead, Kent was asked if he'd be interested in trying an innovative joint capsule shrinkage procedure developed for use in human athletes. It had never been done on dogs, although canine athletes often suffered very similar injuries. The arthroscopic technique uses radio waves that target the damaged, loosened tissue of the joint capsule. The radio waves shrink the tissue, tighten up the joint, and return it to a more normal, close fit. Ken was told that the procedure in people has been shown to last seven or eight years. "In a big dog, that's 80 percent of their life," says Kent.

He feels lucky to have had this chance to try such a noninvasive surgery. Kent was charged only for anesthetic, because Hawk was the first canine patient. Hawk would be in no danger, and if the procedure wasn't successful, they could always re-repair the joint with one of the more established methods.

It took almost three months for them to coordinate the surgery between the surgeons at the hospital currently using the procedure on humans, the veterinary school, and the company that owned the radio-wave machine. Kent saw Hawk's before-and-after pictures on the X rays. "You could see the tissue close around the joint, like your hand closing into a fist—it was amazing!" he says.

Following the surgery, the affected leg was splinted for a week to keep weight off the healing shoulder. Since Hawk's was the first canine procedure, the surgeons didn't know how to predict the healing time. Hawk spent a week in the hospital.

"Everybody loved him," says Ken. "All the medical students waited on him. He's real friendly, he smiles, and he'd walk down the hall and jump up on the counter to get petted." Once he came home, Ken did some massage on the shoulder during Hawk's recovery period, but mostly just leash walked the dog. Hawk was using his leg within a few weeks but was kept on a leash as a precaution. Swimming would have helped speed things up, but Hawk didn't like water. "It was probably three or four weeks before I let him go off-leash, run and play, and do all the normal dog stuff," says Ken. After the fur grew back on his shoulder, Hawk returned to the dog show circuit and resumed a normal life.

Today Ken says Hawk is in his prime at eight years old. "I also have a three-year-old female and she can't keep up with him; he's pretty quick," says Ken. Hawk is also "king dog" around the pair of three-year-old Rhodesian Ridgebacks that belong to Ken's girlfriend. "He's just as young as they are," says Ken.

The surgery has kept Hawk grinning. "He's getting a little gray on the chin," says Ken, "but other than that . . . he keeps up with everybody."

Back Problems

The spine is a string of bones called vertebrae held together by ligaments and cushioned by muscles. The spinal cord travels through a bony canal inside the vertebrae. Disks located between each vertebra are filled with fluid and collagen, a tough fibrous protein. Disks cushion the bone, absorb shock, and allow flexibility. Damage that causes a disk to rupture or slip out of place may injure the spinal cord and cause painful or crippling back problems. Disks that degenerate lose resiliency and encroach on the spinal cord. Injury can happen at any age. Degenerative disk disease starts early in life and gets progressively worse.

Injury to the back can be acute (sudden) due to injury, such as being hit by a car, falling, or just jumping and landing wrong. Even when the dog initially recovers, damage may lead to chronic arthritis as the dog ages. Long-bodied, short-legged dogs such as Dachshunds and Basset Hounds are particularly prone to back problems from injury.

Certain breeds most commonly develop degenerative disk disease, says Lisa Klopp, DVM, an assistant professor of neurology and neurosurgery at the University of Illinois. Degenerative myelopathy is an important disease for geriatric German Shepherds, she says. "It's a very frustrating disease. It's not a painful disease but it is progressive." Older Doberman Pinschers are prone to vertebral malformation and articulation, called Wobbler's syndrome. To a lesser extent, Great Danes may develop Wobbler's, usually before eighteen months of age.

SENIOR SYMPTOMS

Symptoms of back disease or injury vary depending on the location on the spine, and typically affect the dog's ability to function from that point on toward the tail.

- Weak or wobbly gait in the front legs, rear legs, or both
- Hunched posture from pain
- Complete or partial paralysis

Back disease can be devastating. "By the time you see those animals there's often quite a lot of injury to the spinal cord," says Dr. Klopp. The extent of the problem varies from dog to dog. Damage may be reversible or slowed with treatment.

AGE-DEFYING TIPS

When your dog's breed or body conformation makes him more prone to back problems, be alert to early symptoms. Treatment begun early is better able to cure, stop progression, or in some cases prevent the problem altogether.

- Limit extreme jumping for Dachshund-type dogs.
- Keep dogs thin. Weight adds more stress to the back.
- Consider a procedure called laser disk ablation. Now available at Oklahoma State University and elsewhere, tiny needles inserted through the skin of the back into damaged disks allow a laser procedure to vaporize and eliminate the disks without major surgery. It is considered a preventative therapy for problem-prone backs.

TREATING INJURY

Standard treatment for a back injury may be medicine to reduce the inflammation and cage rest for four to six weeks. Surgery that removes the damaged disk and any material impinging on the spinal cord decompresses the injury and aids recovery. Rehabilitation is also required, and dogs may take up to six months to recover.

More recent treatments are more aggressive and encourage gentle exercise such as leash walking, or even better, swim therapy, before and after surgery. Mild physical therapy by itself may offer some improvement and even miraculous relief in a percentage of back-injured dogs.

Dr. Darryl Millis, a surgeon at the University of Tennessee, oversees the first underwater treadmill designed for canine rehabilitation. Other veterinary centers have also made this treatment available to patients. It's especially helpful for back surgery patients, says Dr. Millis. The buoyancy of warm water eases the strain of recovering muscles and also helps relieve pain, which can speed up the rehab process.

Rehabilitation, massage, water therapy, and chiropractic or other physical therapies are absolutely essential for dogs recovering from surgery, especially for the dog with spinal problems, says Signe Beebe, DVM. These patients also require good nutrition to support the healing process. With the proper postsurgery support, Dr. Beebe says, "that animal is going to recover so much more quickly! It's unbelievable."

COMFORT ZONE

Dogs that lose the use of their rear legs may still maintain a quality of life with the help of a wheelchairlike cart. Several companies make custom products—prices vary.

- K-9 Cart Company produces a cart designed by a veterinary orthopedic specialist that is one of the oldest, and available at www.k9carts.com.
- Pet wheelchairs, support slings, paw protectors, and other aids are available at www.doggon.com.
- Wheelchairs for Dogs, www.wheelchairsfordogs.com, is another option.
- Offer a ramp for easy access. The PetSTEP Folding Ramps, available from Drs. Foster and Smith, fold for easy travel and storage, and come in four sizes. Ramps work well, especially for aiding dogs in and out of cars.

DEGENERATIVE DISEASE

Dogs stricken with degenerative myelopathy (DM) suffer from what's thought to be an autoimmune disorder in which the immune system attacks the spinal cord. The result is progressive paralysis. "There are various treatments touted, but my feeling is they don't work," says Dr. Klopp.

"All these dogs eventually stop walking or get to the point where they have a really hard time, and I don't feel like we make much of a dent in that disease."

A holistic treatment developed by Dr. Roger Clemmons, a neurosurgeon at the University of Florida, shows promise for some dogs. A combination of herbs, amino acids, and antioxidants helps reduce the inflammation and protect the nerves to potentially slow the progress of the disease. He reports the natural therapy has stopped progression or caused a remission in up to 80 percent of the patients he's treated.

"With degenerative myelopathy you try to keep the dogs as active as possible," says Dr. Klopp. "Keep them on regular, moderate exercise. Swimming is good. But the bottom line is eventually they won't have enough spinal cord function left to get around."

Wobbler's, also called cervical spondylopathy, is a condition that results from the instability of the neck vertebrae. It develops due to either chronic degenerative disc disease of the last three vertebrae of the neck, or partial dislocation (subluxation) of these vertebrae when the neck is manipulated or moved.

Surgery aims at stabilizing the spine, and removing any ruptured disks, ligaments, or other material compressing the spine. With Wobbler's there will always be a degree of permanent injury, but the amount varies from dog to dog. Dr. Klopp says it's impossible to tell how much the dog may have already compensated for the injury, and surgery that disrupts the balance may, in fact, do more harm than good. "I find it very difficult to predict what animal's going to do what, so I personally don't always treat them surgically," she says.

Changing the dog's lifestyle, especially during the earliest stages of the

---

BOTTOM LINE

Cost of surgical procedures varies in different parts of the country. Combined with rehabilitation and medications, treatment may easily run into the thousands of dollars. "The clients I have would do anything for their animal," says Dr. Beebe. "They say, 'This is my best friend I love.'" Examples of back surgery costs include:

- Standard surgery for canine slipped disk run about $1000 at Oklahoma State University
- Laser disk ablation preventive treatment costs about $400 at OSU

disease, often has a positive effect. "Make them more of a couch potato, stop them from charging after the mailman, or jumping in and out of the back of the truck," says Dr. Klopp. "Put them on a harness, and control the activity. I've had these dogs do very well."

Golden Moments: Free-Wheeling Willy

Willy's early history is a mystery. He was about three years old when he was left in a cardboard box beside a busy street in Los Angeles. The tiny Chihuahua's rear legs didn't work properly, and he had no voice. Not only was Willy paralyzed from the spinal cord injury, he'd also been surgically "debarked." His vocal cords had been cut, and he couldn't complain about his recent injury even if he'd wanted to.

A good Samaritan brought the dog to a local veterinarian's office. Willy spent the next year living in a cage while attempts to reverse his paralysis

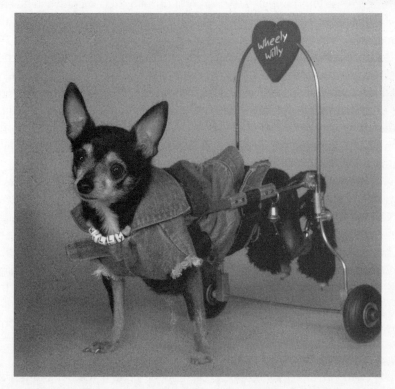

Now that Willy has his wheels, nothing stops him!   *(Photo Credit: Deborah Turner)*

failed. Even worse, the veterinarian and staff weren't able to find a home for the special needs dog, and Willy's euthanasia was eventually scheduled.

"I just felt horrible when I heard the story about the little guy," says Deborah Turner. The owner of a Long Beach pet supply store for seventeen years, Deborah was well known in the area for finding homes for rescue dogs and cats through her business. After learning of Willy's plight, she immediately drove to the city to meet the dog.

"I intended to get him more medical help and place him in a good home," she says. Running her store, caring for the rescue animals and her own personal pets, and other family commitments kept her so busy, she knew Willy's stay could only be temporary. "I envisioned the perfect home would be with a retired person with the time to give him the attention he'd need." Instead, nine years ago Willy came home with her to stay.

The little dog weighed less than two pounds. "He was just a head and two front arms," says Deborah. The rest of his body had atrophied through lack of use. "I thought he was going to be the saddest little guy I had ever seen. But to my shock, this little dog that couldn't bark, couldn't walk, had to drag himself around—he was happy!" Willy literally lit up with excitement when he saw Stevie, the family's silver-tipped Persian. "He dragged himself across the room to play with the cat," says Deborah.

Because of his paralysis, Willy needed help to go to the bathroom. He has normal bowel movements, but can't urinate on his own. "When I got him, he had urine burns because if the bladder filled up, any pressure such as picking him up made him leak," says Deborah. She learned to carry Willy into the bathroom several times a day, hold him over the toilet, and press on his tummy to express the urine. "It's not invasive; it's very easy to do," she says. "Instead of taking him outside, I take him to the toilet."

Willy wanted to be a part of things and didn't let anything slow him down. He pulled himself around the house, dragging his useless rear legs. Deborah wanted to find a way to help the determined dog achieve his goals. "I brought home big helium balloons and attached them to his baby pajamas, trying to get his rear end up off the ground," she says. But Willy was so light, the balloons picked up the entire dog up. "There he hung by his rear end, dangling from the balloons." She was amazed that being airborne never fazed the happy little dog. He stayed perfectly calm and enjoyed the experience.

"Next I tried a skateboard, and then skate wheels. That was ridiculous; there was no control. So I rigged up a baby sack and carried him on my front or back wherever I went," says Deborah.

Life changed for Willy the day Deborah opened one of the pet trade publications she sold in her store and saw the ad for the K-9 Cart Company, a manufacturer of wheelchairs for dogs. It was the perfect solution. Deborah immediately contacted the company and ordered the cart for Willy—it was $200 for a dog his size.

As soon as he was strapped into the wheelchair, Willy was off and running! "He never had to adapt," says Deborah. The little Chihuahua had been waiting for his wheels, and he's not slowed down since. "He walks like any other dog, and he runs as fast as any dog his size," says Deborah.

Today, Willy is a canine celebrity with many television appearances to his credit. He works as a therapy dog in a variety of hospital settings. He serves as a mascot for a group of children called Winners on Wheels, and for the local branch of the Cystic Fibrosis Foundation. He has his own Web site at www.wheelywilly.com and has had two children's books—*How Willy Got His Wheels* and *How Willy Got His Wings*—written about his adventures.

Deborah fully expects Willy to remain healthy for many years to come. "He's big now—he's four pounds! And in nine years, he's never been sick," she says. Other dogs in her pet family have lived to be seventeen and twenty-three, three cats lived to be twenty-four, and one cat is twenty-five and still healthy. She attributes her pets' longevity to a homemade diet. There's no doubt that with the right food, lots of love, and a K-9 Cart, thirteen-year-old Willy will keep rolling right along.

"He's got a wheelchair, but that's no reason to feel sorry for him," says Deborah. "He's the happiest little guy and is just a sweet, docile little dog. He certainly doesn't feel sorry for himself."

Blindness

Blindness can occur at any time in a dog's life, but it tends to develop more often in elderly dogs. Vision loss can be gradual or sudden, complete or partial. Dogs may become blind as a result of injury or, more commonly, as the consequence of an eye disease, such as cataracts, glaucoma, or progressive retinal atrophy (PRA).

"PRA is similar to retinitis pigmentosis in people," says Paul A. Gerding, Jr., DVM. Unlike cataracts or glaucoma, there's no treatment for PRA. The retina progressively degenerates a little at a time. "The cells just start to die," he says. In late-stage disease, the widely dilated pupil makes the eye look very dark.

PRA can be inherited and can affect most breeds but historically has affected Irish Setters, Labradors, Golden Retrievers, Border Collies, Shetland Sheepdogs, Norwegian Elkhounds, and Poodles. "Genetic tests can now detect PRA in the DNA analysis in a lot of breeds," says Dr. Gerding. Tests allow dogs to be diagnosed before they lose their vision. Breeders are able to avoid perpetuating the disease once they know which dogs are affected. And owners can plan to better care for their dog as he loses his sight.

People often remain unaware that dogs have any vision problems at all, because they compensate so well. Loss of sight typically causes problems when they're in unfamiliar surroundings. But at home they know the lay of the house and have mapped it by sight, sound, and scent; they remember each landmark. Owners may suddenly realize there's a problem if they rearrange the furniture, for example.

SENIOR SYMPTOMS

"Dogs will have memorized their own home and yard if they've been there the last five or ten years," says Dr. Gerding. Symptoms of vision loss are therefore more apparent in an unfamiliar environment.

- Bumping into furniture
- Reluctance to navigate stairs or jumps, especially in unfamiliar places
- Becoming clingy, always underfoot
- Snaps when touched unexpectedly
- Reluctant to go outside, especially at night
- Moves more slowly and cautiously
- Pupil of eye stays dilated

A classic sign of PRA is fear of the dark. Dogs do fine in the house, or in the yard during the day, but lose night vision first and become uncomfortable going outside at night.

ACCOMMODATIONS

When blindness is due to cataracts, prompt surgery may restore some vision. But injuries or diseases that cause permanent damage can't be reversed. Blind dogs compensate for the loss by relying more on their other senses, and won't be nearly as concerned about the deficit as the owners, says Harriet Davidson, DVM.

However, the animal's comfort level, safety, and emotional health should be addressed by making necessary accommodations. "Keep all the furniture in one place, and don't move it around too much," says Dr. Davidson. "The animal will memorize the pattern of the house. If the furniture is changed constantly they become a little anxious." It's vital to keep the food and water bowls, the bed, and favorite toys in the same spot, so your dog can always find his belongings. Dr. Davidson also suggests keeping things picked up—for example, don't drop your briefcase in the middle of the hallway—so the dog won't run into objects that are in the way.

Expect that the dog's behavior or personality may change. He will sometimes become more dependent on his owner. "They rely on the owner as a seeing-eye person, instead of a Seeing Eye dog," says Dr. Davidson. "They tend to stand very close and follow you around more." That may be nice because you like to have company, but it may become frustrating when the

```
COMFORT ZONE

Try attaching bells to the collars of other pets in the home, so the blind
dog can more easily find them. It may also help for you to wear a bell, or
speak to announce your presence to avoid startling the dog.
```

dog is always underfoot. "That's a particular concern for elderly folks," says Dr. Davidson, because tripping over the dog could injure both of you. She suggests placing an extra dog bed in the kitchen, for example, and so he has a place to rest that's safely out of the way.

Dogs that have been very social might become standoffish once their vision is gone. "If, for example, you have company to the house for a party, the dog might tend to go to his basket and hide rather than be a part of the party," says Dr. Davidson. "It's because the dog doesn't want to get stepped on and it's just taking care of itself."

A blind dog can become nippy and bite when somebody surprises him. "Be aware of the potential, and warn people—especially children—the dog can't see," says Dr. Davidson. "Make sure that the dog knows they're there before they start petting him." It's not that your dog has suddenly become mean, only that he's startled. It's only fair to warn him, and protect others from an accidental nip.

Keeping the lights turned up can be helpful for PRA dogs with fading vision. "Leave a nightlight on to help the dog navigate around after dark," suggests Dr. Gerding. Also take care to protect him from injury, perhaps blocking off the basement stairs with a baby gate.

Don't let anyone tell you that blind dogs must be put to sleep, says Dr. Gerding. Nothing is farther from the truth. "A blind dog is still a very happy dog," he says.

Golden Moments: Love After Dark

When Katie, a yellow Labrador Retriever, began to go blind between the ages five to seven, her owner never considered that she couldn't still enjoy life. "A dog that suffers rapid vision loss, regardless of the age, typically does have greater problems in switching gears and learning how to get themselves around," says Dr. Gerding. "But dogs that gradually lose vision, whether it be through cataracts or the PRA, remain very good pets." As long as you provide them with food, a yard in which to play, protection, attention, and lots of love, they're happy and they do very well. "They just kind of think the world is dark now," he says. He knows, because Katie is his dog and she has been blind for the past six years.

"I couldn't correct any of Katie's vision changes," says Dr. Gerding. "She's now fifteen years old and she's had a pacemaker for over five years." Like many Labradors, Katie loves to hunt, and blindness didn't stop her. "I've taken her out and hunted her totally blind," says Dr. Gerding. "I'd make sure it was in a clover field, no ditches or roads or holes, and she loved to be out there!"

He says Katie has been a great pet, and still enjoys life to the fullest. "I don't think she looks at anything as being different—it's just dark." He says she's developed set patterns and habits he tries not to break, such as where her bed is, and when she goes out. "She has a system. When she's done outside, she goes through the entire backyard and comes over by the door and is ready to come in, so I get her in right away," he says. "It's a habit, a routine that is very comfortable for her."

Dr. Gerding also has a two-and-a-half-year-old yellow Labrador named Gracie. "Having another dog is sometimes very beneficial to blind dogs," he says. Katie and Gracie run around, jump up and down, and play together all the time. "It's as if she has her own guide dog, because they pick up on each other." If Gracie sees something and barks, Katie can join in. And the younger dog leads the way in their play.

Brain Tumors

Brain tumors are most common in dogs seven to ten years of age, says Lisa Klopp, DVM. Dogs can have quite large tumors and still act normal, but more often they cause behavior changes such as urinary incontinence that may be ascribed to the normal changes of old age. "I see a lot of animals for brain tumors that have been treated for some time for cognizant disorder [senility]," she says. As with any tumor, prompt treatment offers the best hope of remission and/or recovery.

Any animal can get a brain tumor but the Boxer, Golden Retriever, and the Labrador Retriever seem more prone, says Dr. Klopp. Dogs tend to develop certain types of tumor more often than others. "The vast majority of tumors I see in dogs are meningiomas, a tumor of the covering of the brain," she says. Meningiomas are usually quite removable, and the biggest issue is location and how accessible the spot is to the surgeon. Most dogs develop these tumors in the front part of the brain in the olfactory (scenting) region, on the sides or surface, which is relatively easy to reach.

A dog that's ten years old and has had seizures for a month or two but is otherwise healthy may well have a brain tumor, says Dr. Klopp. "A tumor would be the very top of my list." Vascular injury—stroke—may produce similar signs initially, but the symptoms of a stroke typically improve over time; they don't get progressively worse as with a brain tumor.

A general neurological workup may include an MRI, possibly a spinal tap to screen for encephalitis (inflammation of the brain), or an analysis of antibody levels in the blood (titer) for specific diseases. The MRI shows the veterinarian the inside of the brain to determine if it's structurally normal or abnormal. When dogs have symptoms typical of a brain tumor, the MRI will reveal a brain tumor more than 50 percent of the time.

SENIOR SYMPTOMS

Symptoms of a brain tumor are vague and will be variable and depend on what part of the brain is affected. Symptoms may grow progressively worse, or be very suddenly bad.

- Seizure is by far the most common symptom, and is typical of tumors located in the forebrain
- Any behavior change, often similar to cognitive dysfunction symptoms
- Head tilt, weakness, circling, or muscle atrophy on one side of the face are more typical of tumors of the brain stem

---

In most cases, diagnosis stops at that point, although a spinal tap could potentially define some types of tumors. "A spinal fluid analysis is probably not going to be worth the risk if the animal has increased intracranial pressure," says Dr. Klopp. "That could cause brain herniation." Chances of diagnosing a meningiosarcoma from a spinal tap are slim anyway, she says. Depending on what's revealed on the MRI, a tap or titer may or may not be done. The decision is made very much on a case-by-case basis, she says.

Because some brain tumors may be malignant and metastasize—and also, because the age range makes these dogs at high risk for tumors of other types—Dr. Klopp typically does X rays of the chest to make sure there's no cancer. "You don't want to do surgery on a dog that has a chestful of cancer," she says. "You're talking about a pretty big emotional and financial commitment for the owner."

TREATMENT

Once the dog has been diagnosed with a tumor, Dr. Klopp offers them the options. That includes palliative care—keeping the dog comfortable, perhaps with antiseizure medication, until the end—or going after the tumor. Surgery, radiation therapy, and chemotherapy from the cancer arsenal, alone or in combination, may be helpful. Surgery is usually the treatment of choice.

"I don't see people who aren't committed, and they're most comfortable with getting the darn thing out," says Dr. Klopp. "I've done surgery on dogs as old as fourteen."

Brain tumors in dogs do tend to come back. "Probably the longest I've had one [survive surgery] was eighteen months," she says, but she notes that most of her patients are geriatric and die of something else before the tumor returns. "We're buying them time and quality of life rather than curing them. I've never had a client say they wish they hadn't done it. The majority of the time the dogs do very well, and if they don't, owners at least feel like they've done everything they can."

When radiation is used, it can be difficult to avoid damaging normal tissue. An innovative radiation therapy is now available at University of Florida's Evelyn F. and William L. McKnight Brain Institute. The system uses a three-dimensional ultrasound guidance system to pinpoint the tumor's location, and target radiation beams precisely to the tumor, while sparing the surrounding tissue.

With this new technique, pets can be treated in one session of high-dose, precisely targeted X-ray treatment, rather than through repeated sessions over a number of weeks. Radiation therapy on dogs requires anesthetic to keep the pet in the proper position, so the single treatment session avoids the repeated anesthesia that would be a concern in geriatric dogs. The procedure costs roughly the same as for traditional veterinary radiation therapy, but a limited number of animals may be eligible for subsidies or free follow-up care and imaging.

"So far we've done a total of twenty-two animals, including both cats and dogs," says Nola Lester, BVMS, a clinical instructor in radiology with the University of Florida College of Veterinary Medicine. "In some cases we've seen fantastic results and the tumor completely disappears. In others, this is not the case."

BOTTOM LINE

"I'm probably pretty cheap," says Dr. Klopp. "The majority of the cost is the aftercare."

- Most of brain tumor surgeries performed by Dr. Klopp, with follow-up care, run about $2,000.
- Traditional veterinary radiation therapy costs approximately $2,200, and varies in different parts of the country.

Cancer

Dogs suffer from more kinds of cancer than any other domestic animal. The Veterinary Cancer Society says cancer is the leading cause of death in dogs (47 percent), particularly in those over the age of ten. Many canine cancers are the same diseases that people develop. Most commonly, though, dogs suffer from skin cancer (the most common); breast cancer, which accounts for over half the cases; lymphoma, which ranks third, with an incidence of twenty-four cases per 100,000 per year; followed by oral tumors, bone cancer, and testicular cancer.

In the normal process of cell death and replacement, new cells are created in a process called mitosis, in which a cell divides into two identical cells. For unknown reasons, sometimes these new cells mutate into cancer cells that are not identical to the parent cell. Abnormal, fast-growing cancer cells take the place of healthy ones and interfere with normal body functions. The immune system is designed to identify and eliminate abnormal cells, but a breakdown in the system can allow tumors to grow either in one isolated place (called benign), or proliferate throughout the body (malignant).

There are predispositions for cancers in certain breeds or families of dogs, but these tend to occur early in life. In most cases, though, cancers develop in the dog's later years as a result of a lifetime accumulation of injuries or insults, says Barbara Kitchell, DVM. "We're seeing the extremely old geriatrics, like the sixteen-year-old dogs that come in with cancer," she says. "We tend to see more carcinomas in the elderly, maybe because carcinomas appear most often in epithelial tissues." These are the parts of the body, such as skin, lungs, or bladder, which may be impacted by contact with the outside world. That means that damage from the sun or smoke, for example, accumulating over a lifetime, ultimately causes old-age cancer.

SENIOR SYMPTOMS

Signs of cancer vary from type to type, depending on what part of the body is primarily affected. In general, the Veterinary Cancer Society lists ten common signs of cancer.

- Abnormal swelling that persists or continues to grow
- Sores that do not heal
- Weight loss
- Loss of appetite
- Bleeding or discharge from any body opening
- Offensive odor
- Difficulty eating or swallowing
- Hesitation to exercise or loss of stamina
- Persistent lameness or stiffness
- Difficulty in breathing, urinating, or defecating

However, researchers at Purdue University suggest that just as in very old humans, the "oldest-old" among pets may have some cancer resistance. They seldom develop lethal cancers, and their longevity may even be due to this protective ability. Dogs that don't develop cancer until very old probably have a better chance of surviving it because of the same extreme good health that has allowed them to live so long.

DIAGNOSIS

"The key to successful treatment is early diagnosis," says Nichole Ehrhart, VMD. However, care must be taken to ensure that the diagnostic procedure does not make the cancer treatment more difficult. Oftentimes, a suspicious tumor is immediately removed by surgery, and only then sent off for diagnosis. That does save time and cost, says Dr. Ehrhart, but it's vital to do it right. "If you remove something without regard to what it is, oftentimes you disrupt tissue planes that might have been barriers for spread of that tumor," she says. "What could have been a perfectly curable cancer with just surgery alone has been compromised." Without advanced diagnosis, a hurried surgery could result in spreading the cancer so it's harder or even impossible to treat.

The best first step toward diagnosis for external masses is a needle biopsy, says Dr. Ehrhart. "Just put a needle in, take some cells, and look at them on a slide or send them off to a pathologist." This won't always offer a definitive diagnosis, she says, "But it tells you if there are some bad actors in there, and if we should proceed with caution."

When the cancer is on the inside, an ultrasound, X ray, or other imaging technique may be used to locate the tumor. A newer technique called lymphosyntigraphy injects radioactive tracers into the body. Cancer cells tend to absorb these compounds, which makes them easier to locate.

It's best to do a laboratory biopsy on an actual piece of the tumor, and not to rely alone on cells collected in a needle. "Doing a biopsy before removing the mass is one of the wisest things you can do," says Dr. Ehrhart. That allows the doctor not only to determine the kind of cancer, but also to evaluate how advanced the disease is. After that, the veterinarian can better plan an effective treatment. "The best chance you have to surgically cure most cancers is your first cut," says Dr. Ehrhart. She urges pet owners to get that first biopsy done by the pathology lab before removing the whole mass; and if it's cancer, seek referral to a cancer specialist as early as possible.

A diagnosis of cancer can be an emotional experience for the owner. "Cancer is very rarely a physical emergency, but it's almost always a psychological emergency," says Dr. Ehrhart. "That word instills a great amount of fear in people. Making decisions for their own animal when they can't speak for themselves, it's very scary."

It is vital that you are comfortable with and can talk to your doctor, says Dr. Kitchell. "I teach my residents that oncology is practiced in your head and in your heart. It takes both to be good at this job," she says. Beyond that, it's important to sit down and have a heart-to-heart with yourself and with your family. Remember that your dog hasn't a clue anything in his life has changed. He'll understand that you are upset, but he won't know why. He won't be concerned about what the future may hold; he's concerned only about *today*. "We have the ability to make them feel good every single day," says Dr. Ehrhart. "That's our goal in cancer management and treatment."

TREATMENT

Veterinary oncologists design treatments to remove, shrink, or stop the cancer growth, while also protecting the surrounding normal tissue. The same cancer treatments used in people are also used in dogs. These include any one or a combination of surgery, radiation, and chemotherapy. Innovative therapies also may help, usually in combination with a conventional treatment.

"Every patient I treat is an individual," says Dr. Kitchell. "We essentially do a trial in your individual animal, a trial of one. If it works, we keep going. If it makes the animal ill and the quality of life is diminished, we have to get off it."

It's not possible to predict how a given dog will react to a treatment, so there's built-in flexibility, always keeping in mind the owner's goal. "Some clients want to cure the animal of cancer, so I then have the opportunity to give more aggressive therapy, and apply the full gamut of what's available," says Dr. Kitchell. "I also have patients who say, 'He's fourteen, and I want him to live until my kids come home from college to see him in the summer.' But whatever their goal, virtually everybody says, 'I don't want to make him sick in pursuit of treating his cancer.'"

Dr. Ehrhart feels part of her role is to be a client advocate, to discuss options and help people make informed choices. "What's right for you might not be the right choice for the next person," she says. "We will support whatever decision you make."

Surgery

Surgery is the first line of defense against cancer for pets. Removing the tumor can be done with advanced techniques such as lasers and noninvasive arthroscopic technology. It is difficult to achieve a complete cure using surgery alone, however, because leaving behind a single cancer cell opens the possibility of recurrence. In most situations where surgery is used, it is followed by chemotherapy, radiation, or other therapies.

A new treatment technique has particular promise for dogs with bone cancer. Osteosarcoma is an extremely painful, devastating tumor that typically grows near the joint in a leg. The conventional treatment calls for amputation. Removal of the painful leg often makes the dog feel much better, but very athletic dogs may suffer a loss of quality of life. Limb-sparing surgery is an option in which the diseased bone is removed, and replaced with a bone graft, so the dog keeps his leg.

Dr. Ehrhart also offers an experimental procedure called distraction osteogenesis. Once the diseased bone is removed, instead of replacing it with a graft, Dr. Ehrhart induces the dog's body to grow a new bone. The biggest problem with this technique is the slow time it takes for the bone to regenerate. "We can grow bone at the rate of one millimeter per day," says Dr. Ehrhart. "That's extremely fast compared to [the rate at which] a fracture would heal, but from the dog's standpoint it's not fast enough." After the cancerous bone is removed, dogs wear an external brace with wires that go through the skin and bone, and out the other side. A small segment of normal bone is slowly moved each day by adjusting the frame. The owner turns a nut with a wrench three times a day. "You move it a millimeter a day, and that tricks the body into thinking it's trying to heal a fracture," says Dr. Ehrhart. "It's kind of like the carrot before the horse." Eventually the entire defect is replaced with the animal's own bone.

"They look awful [with the brace] but they can walk on it," she explains. "The whole point is to live a normal life, and if they have a median survival of two or three years, I don't want them to be walking around with a brace for four or five months." Dr. Ehrhart is seeking ways to improve the procedure.

Radiation

Surgery may not be practical when the tumor grows in an inaccessible location, such as near vital organs or nerves that also may be damaged, or on the face, where little extra tissue is available. Skin and bone-marrow cancers are particularly treatable with radiation therapy, which aims intense X rays into the malignancy.

There are a couple of concerns with conventional beam radiation, however. The X ray does not discriminate between the cancer and normal tissue, and can damage these areas as well. People treated with radiation therapy for cancers often suffer severe side effects, such as nausea and hair loss, although this is considered rare in dogs. That's because dog tumors treated with this therapy tend to be in the head or neck, and not near the sensitive tissues of the lungs or intestines, as is often the case with people. Some dogs may temporarily lose their appetite or shed whiskers. Radiation cures up to 80 percent of some kinds of cancers.

Some of the newest linear accelerators (radiation machines) are designed to better target the tumor while sparing normal tissue. These technologies may incorporate CAT scanners to help "see" the tumor in three dimensions and better plan the treatment. Washington State University has a linear accelerator that features a computerized forty-leaf collimator that works like the iris on a camera to pinpoint the tumor with the X-ray beam. The head of the machine rotates around the pet's body and adjusts the dose of radiation as it moves.

Radiation treatment requires anesthetic, which involves risks that are of greater concern, especially for senior dogs. Pets won't hold still for the radiation to be targeted, and they require repeated anesthesia for a series of treatments.

One of the newest radiation therapies addresses both anesthesia concerns and the toxicity issue. The University of Florida veterinarians and scientists offer stereotactic radiosurgery using a specially designed medical linear accelerator in conjunction with a three-dimensional ultrasound guidance system. The therapy is able to target radiation beams precisely to tumors (and spare normal tissue), and uses a onetime extremely high radiation dose instead of repeated sessions over a number of weeks. That means animal patients receive a single dose of anesthesia rather than several.

So far, about twenty-two animals have been treated, says Nola Lester, BVMS. In some cases, the tumor has completely disappeared, and in others the procedure is not as effective. Dr. Lester says they are still in the early stages of figuring out what works best. The procedure costs roughly the same amount as traditional veterinary radiation therapy.

Chemotherapy

Chemotherapy uses cell-poisoning (cytotoxic) drugs to address cancers that have spread throughout the body. Drugs may be given as pills, injections, or intravenously. Often chemo is prescribed following cancer surgery, to help "catch" any errant cells that were missed. Most of these drugs are adapted from human medicine, and they may be used alone or in various combinations. Some work better than others for different cancers, and the price ranges from extremely expensive to quite reasonable.

There is no such thing as a "standard" chemotherapy treatment, says Dr. Kitchell. Everybody has their favorite combinations or scheduling, and even then, cost factors may influence the treatment choice. "It's amazing how sometimes you're so surprised," she says. "You know this isn't an optimum therapeutic pathway, but *wow!* is this animal doing great on it! When you treat cancer, you see miracles all the time."

If the first drug you try doesn't work, it's not the end of the world. "Chemotherapy is not like jumping off a cliff," says Dr. Ehrhart. "You can do a reduced dose the next time or change drugs. There are many choices."

Age adds a level of complexity to the therapy because elderly dogs lose reserve capacity in the liver and kidneys, where the drugs used to treat cancer have to be metabolized. "We have to be especially careful with geriatric patients when we try to treat them," says Dr. Kitchell. "When you treat with cancer drugs, there are risks. You can't predict who's going to be supersensitive."

BOTTOM LINE

- Bone grafts may run as high as $3,000
- Radiation therapy series cost about $2,200

OTHER OPTIONS

Besides the standard three treatments, some cancers respond to innovative therapies such as cryosurgery, in which localized, shallow tumors are frozen and destroyed using (usually) liquid nitrogen. Cryosurgery is particularly helpful on skin cancers of the face.

In photodynamic therapy (PDT), sensitizing agents similar to chlorophyll, which the cancer absorbs, are injected into the dog's body. The cancer is then treated with laser light. The energy released within the sensitized cells kills the tumor but leaves normal tissue untouched. PDT is particularly useful against certain skin cancers, oral tumors, and bladder tumors.

Heat therapy (hyperthermia) basically cooks the cancer to kill it, using sound waves that penetrate the body at specific depths and dimensions. Ongoing studies in hyperthermia cancer applications in animals continue at University of Illinois and North Carolina State University—Raleigh.

Gene therapy is the latest frontier in veterinary cancer treatments. Treatments for the most part remain experimental. For example, studies on genetically engineered tumor vaccines designed to target mouth cancers are being conducted by E. Gregory MacEwen, VMD, ACVIM, and his team at the University of Wisconsin.

Nutrition

Supporting the dog with good nutrition, while he is receiving other treatments, is vital, says Susan Wynn, DVM, a holistic veterinarian and executive director of the Georgia Holistic Veterinary Medical Association and of the Veterinary Botanical Medicine Association. "We think homemade diets really help them feel better. It's not to say that [commercial] cancer diets aren't good, but sometimes putting them on a homemade diet gives them kind of a boost—we don't really know why."

Studies by Dr. Gregory Ogilvie at Colorado State and others show that cancer changes the way the body uses food. Oftentimes dogs with cancer lose weight even though they continue to eat. "Called cachexia, that means the tumor is diverting energy toward the growth of the tumor instead of building up the body," says Sheila McCullough, DVM. Dogs with a variety of malignancies—ranging from lymphoma and osteosarcomas to thyroid carcinomas and mammary cancers—were screened. "They all had very similar metabolic abnormalities," says Debbie Davenport, DVM, an internist and director for special education for Hill's Pet Nutrition. "Unless you changed their diet, even if you treated their cancers in what appeared to be an effective way, you couldn't make those metabolic abnormalities change."

By changing the diet, doctors attempt to outwit the cancer, and holistic veterinarians say dogs eating homemade diets enjoy a better quality of life. It's important, though, to design any homemade diet with the help of a veterinary nutritionist to avoid making the dog even sicker. The Web site www.petdiets.com is run by veterinary nutritionists who can help you and your veterinarian design an appropriate recipe. "I recommend one that's about 50 percent poultry or fish, 50 percent veggies, plus appropriate vitamins and minerals," says Dr. Wynn. In addition, she includes fish oils for their antioxidant properties, as well as turmeric and garlic. "That's not for flavor," she explains. "Turmeric (*Curcuma longa*) inhibits tumor growth and metastasis, reduces side effects of chemotherapy, and increases the action of some chemotherapy agents." How much to offer in the food depends on the individual dog, and requires veterinary supervision.

In conjunction with Hill's Pet Foods, Dr. Ogilvie's group has worked to create a commercial diet designed to counter the metabolic changes caused by cancer. Tumors thrive on glucose (blood sugar), but may have trouble using fat for energy. Prescription Diet n/d has a unique nutrient profile. Among other things, it is relatively low in simple carbohydrates, and relatively high in DHA, a polyunsaturated fatty acid thought to prevent the growth and spread of tumors.

To date, there have been three hundred dogs involved in clinical trials testing the commercial diet. "In the lymphoma and radiation therapy patients, the results have really been dramatic," says Dr. Davenport. "We can actually prolong life, prolong remission time, and even more important, improve quality of life. Since the publication of the dog data, there have been a series of publications in people using a similar nutritional profile showing the same result. It's one of those times that we developed a nutritional technology that's now been adopted by the human medical community."

Alternative Therapies

Holistic practitioners often recommend an integrated approach to dealing with cancer. Adjunct therapies that incorporate herbs and supplements may help counteract or diminish side effects of cancer treatments, or boost the action of radiation or chemotherapy. They also help support the dog during the healing and recovery period following surgery, says Signe Beebe, DVM. "For example, you can use Traditional Chinese Medicine to improve the blood cell count that has a tendency to drop as a side effect of the strong radiation or chemotherapy," she says.

"Inositolhexaphosphoric acid, or phytate, is contained in grains like barley," says Dr. Wynn. "You get it as the extract called IP6 from health food stores." There have been studies indicating IP6 may help control the spread of tumors. Dr. Wynn says IP6 may also have a preventive role in addition to helping as an antioxidant.

Green tea may also inhibit tumor growth and angiogenesis—the formation of blood vessels that feeds the cancer and allows the tumors to spread. Dogs can be given the brewed tea to drink, or the leaves can be added to canned food. Certain mushrooms, such as Reishi, shiitake, and Maitake mushrooms, are also known to stimulate immunity and fight tumors, says Dr. Wynn. Most are available only as dried products or extracts from holistic veterinary sources.

Dogs tend to have a limited tolerance for accepting medicines. Dr. Wynn suggests creating a first, second, and third group of medicines or treatment choices. That way your dog can benefit from the most helpful ones first. "My first tier is a natural diet, with antioxidants and fish oil," she says. After that, if the dog tolerates more, a second tier might be IP6 and mushrooms. It depends on the animal.

PROGNOSIS

Prognosis depends on the individual animal, the kind of cancer, and the type of treatment. As with any chronic illness, quality of life is paramount. "There's only a certain amount of time that any of us has on the planet," says Dr. Kitchell. "So you want to make every day that animal has a good day, a golden day." Cures are often possible, she says, but cancer is virtually impossible to cure after a relapse. A recurrence means that despite the treatment, the dog will ultimately lose the war.

"If the cancer is getting tougher, then we have to toughen up our treatment approach to try and get it back under control," says Dr. Kitchell. "Anytime along that pathway, the client is free to say, 'Enough is enough.' Usually by that point, treatment has given people the time they need to adjust to the loss."

AGE-DEFYING TIPS

There is no absolute way to prevent cancer, but there are steps you can take to reduce risk factors for your dog.

- Spaying and neutering dogs at an early age decreases the risk of mammary cancer in females, and prostate cancer in male dogs. Dogs spayed before their first heat cycle will have a relative risk of 0.05 percent for mammary cancer, whereas those with one heat cycle have an 8 percent risk, and two or more cycles increase their risk to 26 percent risk.
- Dogs with white, thin-haired abdomens are at risk for sun-induced cancer. Protect them from sunburn with a T-shirt, human or canine sunscreen products, or by preventing outside exposure during the brightest time of the day.
- Secondhand smoke and chlorine in drinking water increases the risk of bladder cancer in dogs. Protect dogs from exposure to these carcinogens.
- Obesity increases the risk of cancer. Keep dogs thin.

Golden Moments: Scout's Lucky Break

Five years ago, Scout the Standard Poodle got lucky. The lovable black dog lived in Oklahoma, and managed to escape her dog run. After being missing for twenty-four hours, she returned home with a broken leg. Her owners took her to the veterinarian and asked that Scout be put to sleep.

The veterinarian took one look at the happy, tail-wagging sweet dog—and couldn't do it. Instead, she had the owners sign over their rights to the dog, and then the veterinarian put a pin in her broken leg and found her a new home through Poodle rescue services. Janine and Barry Adams, who already had another black Poodle named Kramer, welcomed Scout into their home and hearts.

"Scout is an extremely optimistic, happy-happy dog," says Janine. "We lucked out! She charmed a vet into saving her life."

Although Kramer had many health problems and was a serious dog, happy-go-lucky Scout remained "ultrahealthy," says Janine. "Scout waited until Kramer got healthy before she got sick," she says.

In February 2001, Janine was attending the annual February Westminster Kennel Club Dog Show when she learned that eight-year-old Scout was sick. "It looked like a bacterial infection of the middle ear—her ears were twitching," says Janine. Scout got better with antibiotics but still wasn't completely well, and her blood work didn't return to normal. "She was becoming increasingly anemic," says Janine.

Janine's veterinarian found and removed a mammary tumor on Scout, which turned out to be benign, but two days later Janine noticed blood in the dog's urine. "She peed red," says Janine, "so the assumption was cystitis." More antibiotics were prescribed, but there was no improvement. By this time, Scout's ears were quivering and twitching nonstop. "We decided to do an ultrasound to look for bladder stones," says Janine.

Instead, they found an orange-size tumor growing out of Scout's left kidney. It pressed on the bundle of nerves that triggered the ear twitching. On March 23, Scout's kidney and the tumor were removed. She was in the hospital a couple of days, and returned home on March 25th—her buddy Kramer's ninth birthday. The good news was that for a change Kramer was feeling terrific.

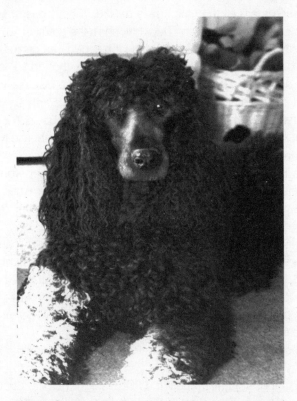

When Scout was diagnosed with cancer, natural therapies kept her feeling good. *(Photo Credit: Janine Adams)*

The bad news was that Scout had cancer. Janine and Barry learned that the tumor was a very fast, aggressive sarcoma. The surgeon removed as much of it as possible, but the tumor was so large that part of it had entered the abdomen.

"The scare, of course, is the cancer will come back. Apparently it's almost bound to come back," says Janine. "But for right now, she's feeling great! She was running around in the park this morning like a puppy chasing her ball, jumping around like a bucking bronco."

In the meantime, Janine has worked with a team of veterinarians to care for Scout and maintain her quality of life. Dr. Kruesi, a holistic veterinarian in Vermont, evaluates blood tests and uses the results to design an appropriate homemade diet, supplemented with vitamins and minerals to keep Scout healthy. "We're trying to build her immune system, using things like shark cartilage, IP6, and Essiac tea to stop any new growths," says Janine.

On the local front, Dr. Karen Mateyak at Animal Kind Veterinary Hospital works with Janine and Scout. "The people at our clinic just love my dogs, because they see them all the time," says Janine. "Scout goes behind the reception desk and they baby her. They think she's the greatest."

Janine says she really hasn't thought of her dogs as senior citizens yet. "They're ill, but not infirm. Scout does have arthritis, though." The orthopedic pin in her leg has caused some degenerative joint disease in her knee. They've not had to make accommodations for Scout's arthritis yet, but plan to do so when they move from New York back to St. Louis. "Our old house has a big oak staircase. The plan is to put carpeting on the staircase for her, so she has traction if she tears down the steps."

Exercise helps keep the dog active and healthy. Scout won't retrieve— very unusual for a Poodle—but she loves to chase Kramer when he's retrieving. "That works out nicely," says Janine. "Thankfully Kramer doesn't mind being chased."

On July 6, 2001, Janine and Barry learned that Scout's cancer had returned. The surgeon told them that the new tumor was inoperable, and that they should enjoy the month or so they had left with Scout. They did.

Luck brought Scout into their life, and she returned the favor by teaching her owners how to enjoy life to the fullest. Janine says every single day became a cherished treasure.

Scout fooled the specialists and outlived all their predictions. She enjoyed a high quality of life and remained pain-free for seven months following her initial March diagnosis, right up until the last week of her life. On October 16, Barry and Janine gave their sweet Scout the greatest gift of all—a peaceful, loving death.

Cataracts

Dogs suffer from cataracts more than any other species. It can be an inherited condition in certain breeds, especially Cocker Spaniels and Poodles, and some puppies are born with cataracts. Most times, though, dogs suffer from "old age" cataracts that develop with age.

SENIOR SYMPTOMS

Signs of cataracts develop slowly and may not be obvious until suddenly you notice the dog can't see. Watch for:

- Cloudy lens within the eye
- Impaired vision characterized by bumping into furniture, or cautious movements, especially in strange surroundings

---

Almost all dogs over the age of five years begin to have some degree of normal cloudiness to the lens of the eye, due to nuclear sclerosis, says Paul A. Gerding, Jr., DVM. Dogs can see through this cloudiness without a problem. Cataracts, though, cause vision loss.

Cataracts are caused by changes in the clear lens of the eye that turn the lens cloudy and opaque. A cataract may affect only a small part of the lens, and the dog can compensate by seeing "around" the area. Other times, the entire lens turns white, and the dog loses vision until eventually she becomes blind. The longer these cataracts "mature," the more difficult it becomes to treat them successfully.

"The rapidly developing cataracts are often attributed to diabetes," says Dr. Gerding. That happens when the protein in the lens of the eye is damaged by metabolic changes caused by diabetes.

Patients diagnosed by general-practice veterinarians may then be referred to veterinary ophthalmologists. "Surgery is the only way to treat cataracts," says Harriet Davidson, DVM.

TREATMENT

If the dog has other health complications, such as heart disease, anesthesia could be a potential risk, and so more care must be taken. But advanced age does not preclude cataract surgery. "A fifteen- to seventeen-year-old dog who's in good health is certainly a good candidate for cataract surgery," says Dr. Gerding.

Cataracts typically cause inflammation in the eye, and that may need to be addressed before surgery can take place. Your own vet will often prescribe the drops, which can be either steroidal drugs or nonsteroidal, depending on the dog's situation. "If an animal is diabetic you typically don't use steroids," says Dr. Gerding. "Once the inflammation checks out fine, we schedule the surgery."

Surgery uses a process called phacoemulsification, which is ultrasonic fragmenting of the lens by sound waves, followed by the removal of the lens. It's the same procedure used in people, says Dr. Gerding. A hollow needle inserted into the eye sends vibrations into the lens. The pieces are vacuumed out through the same hollow needle.

Removing the cloudy lens restores sight, but it typically leaves the dog farsighted unless artificial lenses are inserted. "They never have the same vision they had as a puppy," says Dr. Davidson. "But they do get their vision back so they can play and navigate their area and not run into things. It improves their quality of life," says Dr. Davidson.

"Usually both eyes are involved, and we highly recommend doing both eyes at once," says Dr. Gerding. The cost isn't much different for one eye or both, so it's more economical and requires only one session of anesthesia to do them at the same time.

Recovery time varies. "If they're diabetic usually they go home that same day," says Dr. Gerding, so that insulin and other treatment can be maintained. If they're not diabetic, they go home the next morning.

"The healing phase is most critical the first couple of weeks after surgery, but we are real cautious for four to six weeks before they resume total physical activities," says Dr. Gerding. Dogs typically develop more eye inflammation after surgery than people do, and need eyedrops to control that.

Dogs are also a bit different from people in how they react after the surgery. Says Dr. Gerding, "Their eyes will see right away, but how they're interpreting sight in their brain will be variable. Some dogs wake up from surgery and are immediately visual. Others may take several days or so before they're truly responding. We're not sure why that is, but I think that has to do with the effects of the anesthesia."

"It's a very expensive surgery and it's not without risks," says Dr. Davidson. "If the owner chooses not to have cataract surgery, it's not unkind to let the animal live blind." She says a blind dog can still be a wonderful pet, and if her owner makes accommodations to keep her safe, she can do very well.

It's important to continue routine eye checks on dogs with cataracts, though. Cataracts can lead to other conditions such as inflammation of the eye (uveitis), which can lead to glaucoma. The veterinarian can monitor the dog's eyes for uveitis, and if necessary, treat it using anti-inflammatory eyedrops.

BOTTOM LINE

Cataract surgery typically costs about $1000 per eye, says Dr. Gerding. "It's highly recommended to replace their lens with artificial implants, but sometimes you can't get them in," he says. "The implants run about $200 each, so if they're not used, it would be that much less per eye."

Golden Moments: Gambling on Heidi

When Heidi developed diabetes at age eight, owners Tina and Bob Horton had their hands full simply saving the dog's life. She'd finally recovered with regular insulin therapy and seemed back to normal when Tina noticed a drastic behavior change in the lovable Greyhound-Doberman mix. "She'd hang her head down. She would sit and stare up at the walls. She loved to ride in the car, but then didn't want to go in the car anymore. She couldn't find anything—she couldn't *see* anything," says Tina.

Heidi had developed cataracts and was almost blind. Cataracts often develop in diabetic dogs when the lens protein is damaged by metabolic changes caused by the diabetes.

Tina told Bob that after spending so much money on the diabetes, she just couldn't let the dog go blind. Heidi's primary veterinarian, Dr. Louis Cronin of the Dwight Veterinary Clinic, in Dwight, Illinois, told them about the veterinary ophthalmologists available in Champaign.

At the end of November, they took Heidi down for pre-evaluation with ophthalmologist Dr. Paul Gerding and ophthalmology resident Dr. Teresa Tucci at the Veterinary Teaching Hospital's Comparative Ophthalmology Service. "We should have gone earlier than we did, but we waited six months," says Tina.

First, they had to raise the money. Tina says she's not much of a gambler, but she took $50 to the riverboat. "I said, *'Please, dear God, let me win for Heidi's sake . . . '* and I did! I did! That paid for a big part of her cataract surgery." The Hortons' children made up the difference. They gave no Christmas presents to each other that year. "We had the Heidi fund, and everybody put the Christmas money in, and that's how we paid for the cataract surgery," says Tina.

The surgery was scheduled for the 8th of December. The Hortons took Heidi to the clinic the day before and were to be called the day after the procedure. But when Dr. Gerding began the call with "I'm so sorry," Tina's heart skipped a beat—she thought Heidi must have died under the anesthesia. Because of her advanced age and diabetes, Tina knew Heidi was at greater risk for the anesthesia. She was relieved to learn nothing was wrong with Heidi—but the phacoemulsifier machine was not working properly. The doctors advised postponing the surgery for another week to allow time to correct the machine.

The Hortons brought Heidi home. Being at the clinic was complicated by the fact that Heidi didn't want to eat there, and they had to force-feed her. She also was reluctant to eat at home. "If I'm not home she won't eat," says Tina. She learned that the dog would eat at home, though, if Tina sang to her. "I made my own songs up, my own melody, waltzes and polkas, and she would come to me and start eating," says Tina.

A week later, Heidi returned for the rescheduled surgery. Once again, though, Dr. Gerding explained they were not able to remove the cataracts with the phacoemulsifier. This time, because Heidi's cataracts were so mature (dense), the machine wouldn't be effective.

Instead they used a different but effective procedure that required a larger incision. This standard treatment had been used prior to the availability of the phaco unit.

The prognosis was mixed. One of Heidi's eyes came through the surgery very well and likely would regain vision. But they weren't sure about the other eye, because the retina had detached due to all the inflammation. Although the medical treatment greatly improved the comfort of the eye by removing much of the inflammation, the surgery might not restore vision.

"We picked her up on a Saturday," says Tina. "She wore a lampshade collar, and she hated that thing." The Elizabethan collar restraint kept the dog from further injuring her healing eyes by pawing at them. "She was slinging and banging it at everything, and was completely obnoxious! We had to leave it on for almost two weeks." Tina was also instructed not to let Heidi off the leash.

Just before Christmas snow hit, and the drifts were enormous. "I had to walk her through the snow even in the middle of the night. She couldn't see anything," says Tina. "She would take this lampshade and use it as a snow shovel, and shove the snow around. Heidi was completely frustrated."

At the checkup Tina was told both eyes were healing nicely. She was given two different kinds of eyedrops to administer every morning and night to Heidi's eyes. "Even though we weren't sure about vision outcome in the eye that was most inflamed, it was still very important to be treating it," says Dr. Gerding. The drops helped counter the inflammation, eased discomfort, and was a quality-of-life issue for Heidi. Tina continued to medicate both eyes with the drops.

The combination of the eye medicine, the insulin, and the detested snow put a lot of strain on Heidi—and on her owners. The ninety-mile drive in the snow to the clinic for each checkup made it even worse.

At recent checkups, Dr. Gerding says they were very surprised how much Heidi had improved in the most inflamed eye. Somehow the retina has reattached, and now Heidi has vision in both eyes.

But despite the hardship, Tina says she would do it over again in the blink of an eye. "I think it's a miracle; she's my miracle dog!" says Tina.

Heidi no longer demands a song before eating. She once again looks forward to her daily walk in the nearby village park. "She still tries to run, but

---

NURSE ALERT!

Following cataract surgery, dogs need to receive eyedrops four to six times a day for at least two weeks, to control potential eye inflammation. Even without surgery, cataracts may predispose a dog's eye to inflammation that will require drops.

she's getting arthritis in her hind legs," says Tina. "I have arthritis myself and I take glucosamine, so I pop a pill down her, too, and it helps."

Tina knows that big dogs don't live very long, and at fourteen, the time Heidi has left with them is precious. Tina says the love they've given Heidi has been returned in full. "We always laugh and say Heidi has nine lives. She has a few more to go, I think."

Constipation

Difficult or less-frequent-than-normal passage of dry, hard feces is called constipation. The colon is designed to pull moisture from waste, and if feces stays in the colon too long, it becomes painful to move the waste out of the body.

Elderly dogs may lose muscle tone and have more difficulty evacuating their bowels. Reduced exercise also is often a cause. Older dogs may be more reluctant to go outside during extremes of weather—very hot or very cold temperatures may prompt them to "hold" it for longer periods, and develop constipation.

Constipation isn't a problem specific to old dogs, but it can certainly affect them. A condition of intact old male dogs called perineal hernia causes similar signs. The male hormone testosterone has been shown to have a significant role in the weakening of the perineal muscles. This allows the intestine to protrude through the muscle wall on either side of the anal opening, right beneath the tail.

The perineal hernia often traps feces within its pouch and prevents the material from leaving the body, and affected dogs often strain and show other signs of constipation even when defecating, says Colin Burrows, BvetMed. Surgery is necessary to correct the defect. Surgically altering male and female dogs at a young age prevents nearly all of these concerns.

TREATMENT

Most cases of constipation won't need veterinary care. Adding cow's milk to the dog's food, or a fiber source such as nonflavored Metamucil, bran cereal, or canned pumpkin, often gets things moving naturally again. For small dogs, add one teaspoon of Metamucil twice daily to the food, and two to three teaspoons twice a day for larger dogs. For canned pumpkin or squash, add one half teaspoon to a small dog's food or two tablespoons to large dog's food. Most dogs like the flavor.

SENIOR SYMPTOMS

Older dogs commonly suffer from intermittent bouts of constipation. It's important to keep an eye on your dog's deposits, so you can get her help if needed. Symptoms include:

- Straining without passing stool
- Dry, hard stool with dark brown liquid

If that doesn't work, the veterinarian may need to become involved. Suppositories, enemas, or laxatives can be required in more serious cases, as well as fluid therapy if the dog has become dehydrated.

A good senior diet also helps keep your dog regular. These are not necessarily higher in fiber, but they may contain different ingredients that help keep the intestinal lining healthy, says Dan Carey, DVM.

AGE-DEFYING TIPS

Preventing constipation is based on common sense, says Sarah K. Abood, DVM. Pay attention to your dog's environment, and make adjustments accordingly.

- When it's hot out, make sure there's plenty of water.
- Offer regular meals. A disruption in the schedule can throw off the dog's system.
- Encourage regular exercise.
- Keep the fur beneath the tail on longhaired dogs trimmed to prevent mats, which can cause external blockage that interferes with defecation.
- Feed a "senior" diet. Most include the right amount and kinds of fiber to ward off constipation.

Simply adding extra fiber to give more bulk but no energy is not fair to the intestinal tract. "It's like somebody at the end of a marathon being told, here, carry this," says Dr. Carey. Moderately fermentable fiber, such as beet pulp and rice bran, can be broken down by the "good" bacteria to release energy for itself and for the lining of the intestine.

Cushing's Disease

Cushing's disease, or hyperadrenocorticism, was named for the doctor who first described this syndrome in people. It is a common metabolic disorder of dogs in which the adrenal gland secretes an excess of cortisol, says Richard Nelson, DVM, an internist at the University of California—Davis. "We see quite a bit of Cushing's disease in older dogs here. It usually occurs around eight to ten years of age."

Cortisol affects the metabolism of carbohydrates, proteins, and fats. It also suppresses the body's inflammatory and immune responses. Too much secreted into the system reduces the body's resistance to bacteria and viruses. Beagles, Boston Terriers, Boxers, Dachshunds, and Toy and Miniature Poodles appear to have an increased risk for the condition. The disease is a progressive one that is slow and insidious.

There are different forms of the disease. "The most common form affects the pituitary gland at the base of the brain," says Dr. Nelson. In the pituitary form of Cushing's disease, a tiny and otherwise benign tumor causes the pituitary to overstimulate the adrenal gland. Smaller-breed dogs tend to get tumors of the pituitary gland, says Dr. Jana Gordon, a resident in internal medicine at the University of Illinois.

About 20 percent of Cushing's disease is the adrenal form, in which tumors develop on the adrenal glands themselves, says Dr. Nelson. "The adrenal glands are located down next to the kidney, one on each side, little tiny kidney-bean shaped organs about an inch in length. Sometimes you'll get a cancer that secretes too much cortisol."

SENIOR SYMPTOMS

Cushing's disease is associated with signs very similar to those of diabetes and kidney failure, says Dr. Nelson. All three are "old dog" diseases, which can make diagnosis confusing. How many symptoms or combinations of signs you see depends on the dog, the severity of the disease, and how long it's been going on.

- Increased appetite
- Increased thirst
- Excessive urination
- Lethargy
- Symmetrical hair loss on the body
- Progressive potbelly
- Wasting or weakening of legs
- Skin discoloration and thinning

Neurologic signs may include:

- Pacing
- Circling
- Drunken walk
- Head pressing
- Seizures

Larger-breed dogs are more likely to develop tumors of the adrenal gland, says Dr. Gordon. Yet another form of the disease can be induced by the overuse of cortisone-type medications, which are often used to control itchy skin conditions.

Complications of Cushing's disease include increased risk of infection, high blood pressure, congestive heart failure, pancreatitis, diabetes, and blood-clotting abnormalities.

Blood tests evaluate the adrenal gland function by measuring the amounts of circulating hormones when the dog is at rest, and in response to adrenal gland stimulating and suppressing drugs. Treatment depends on where the tumor is located.

TREATMENT

The pituitary form of the disease is treated with oral medication that controls cortisol secretion from the adrenals. Lysodren (mitotane), also known as o,p,-DDD, is most often prescribed, and it works in almost all cases. It is structurally related to the insecticide DDT, and is cytotoxic. That is, it destroys the adrenal gland cells. Typically, mitotane is given for the rest of the dog's life, and quickly reverses many of the symptoms within days to weeks.

Ketoconazole (Nizoral) is an alternative drug treatment for dogs that do not respond well to mitotane. It inhibits adrenal hormone production and is considered less toxic than mitotane. It is not FDA approved, but use in dogs is common and is considered accepted practice.

Surgical removal of the affected gland is the treatment of choice for the adrenal form of Cushing's, says Dr. Nelson. When the tumor is on only one gland, removing that gland cures the disease. In dogs that do not respond well to any medication, both glands may be removed, followed by oral medication to replace the missing hormones.

A new supplement on the market, S-Adenosylmethionine (SAMe) is a nutraceutical antioxidant that may be helpful in Cushing's patients with liver complications. A commercial S-Adenosylmethionine supplement (Denosyl SD4) has been demonstrated to improve liver function in these pets.

Treatment for Cushing's disease reverses the symptoms and improves the dog's quality of life. It helps the dog live an average of about eighteen months longer, says Dr. Gordon.

NURSE ALERT!

Dogs diagnosed with Cushing's disease usually require medication for the rest of their lives. Mitotane is toxic and requires careful handling. Owners should wash their hands after giving the drug.

Deafness

Deafness is a failure to respond to sound stimuli. Dogs rely on hearing to stay connected with their owners and the world around them. Many normal dog behaviors are interconnected with hearing, so these behaviors begin to change as the dog loses the ability to hear. "When it's a gradual change, the owner may be unaware of that for some time," says George M. Strain, DVM.

Puppies can be born deaf when there are problems with the auditory nerve that transmits sound from the inner ear to the brain. Called sensorineural hearing loss, the condition may be inherited, and is more likely in breeds such as Dalmatians and Jack Russell Terriers.

Other conditions may cause degrees of hearing loss over the dog's life. Drug toxicities such as gentamicin sulfate (an antibiotic) can produce hearing loss because they're toxic to the nerve cells of the ear, says Dr. Strain. There are almost two hundred medications that can be toxic to hearing and cause deafness. "Those drugs usually have to be given systemically [swallowed or injected], rather than topically as eardrops, to produce this effect," says Dr. Strain. He says drops are normally not a problem.

The most common type of deafness is age-related hearing loss, called presbycusis, which develops when the internal hearing structures of the ear gradually degenerate. "It may be slow and progressive or rapid; there's no way to predict that," says Dr. Strain. Toxicities and sound trauma can increase the rate of the normal process of presbycusis. Hunting dogs often lose hearing due to the trauma of gunfire.

SENIOR SYMPTOMS

Behavior changes are the most common symptoms of hearing loss in dogs.

- Increased sleeping. "The dog used to be waiting at the door when you got home because he heard the car coming. Instead the dog's still asleep on the sofa, where it's not supposed to be," says Dr. Strain.
- Voice commands are often ignored.
- Decreased barking, voice that sounds "odd."
- More easily startled.
- Snapping. "If they're startled, sometimes they'll reflexively bite before they have time to recognize that this is not really a threat," says Dr. Strain.

"There is a reflex that contracts the two tiniest muscles in the body inside the middle ear," says Dr. Strain. That is a self-protective reflex that acts like a biological muffler—by contracting those muscles the sound that gets to the inner ear is reduced. "Before a dog barks, that muscle contracts so the dog's own vocalization doesn't damage his hearing," says Dr. Strain. If there's pain associated with a loud noise, dogs have enough sense to move away, but a percussive sound such as gunfire happens too fast. Says Dr. Strain, "I see a lot of Labradors, champion field trial dogs, whose range to respond to signals and whistles or calls is cut in half. That is a cumulative hearing loss, and the ear does not recover from that."

ACCOMMODATIONS

Since most hearing loss is associated with age, these older dogs often have other age-related problems such as arthritis. Hunting dogs and field trial dogs may be retired from competition and, like other pet dogs, continue to enjoy a good quality of life.

Hearing loss can affect the way you interact with your dog, and some accommodations will help maintain the bond you share. Deaf dogs typically begin to rely more on their other senses, such as sight, and frequently learn to respond to hand signals rather than voice commands. You just have to get their attention first.

For example, deaf dogs are often taught to respond to the porch light flashing on and off, rather than being called to come in. Although they can't hear, deaf dogs can still feel vibration, so a slammed door or stomped foot may work as a signal. It's particularly important to give the deaf dog some sort of warning of your presence to avoid a startle/bite reflex.

Some dogs lose hearing only in certain ranges. High-pitched "dog whistles" might still be detectable by certain dogs. In homes with multiple pets, animals with hearing loss often take their cues from other animals in the household. "If one animal suddenly gets up and starts barking, the deaf one will get up and move around, too," says Dr. Strain.

Besides quality-of-life concerns, deafness becomes a safety issue for outdoor animals. If they don't hear the car coming, for example, they may not be able to avoid being hit.

HEARING AIDS

Dogs with some types of hearing loss may benefit from a hearing aid. Remember, though, that a hearing aid is an amplifier. It won't help if the dog has no hearing function left. But those that are simply "hard of hearing" may be candidates.

A number of efforts have been made over the years to create viable commercial hearing aids for dogs. The problem is that the dog's ear canal is shaped differently from a human's, and it's been difficult to find something that not only fits, but that a dog will tolerate. "It seems that smaller-breed animals tolerate them better than large-breed dogs," says Dr. Strain.

Human hearing aids are fitted by making a mold of the ear canal. The canine ear canal is an L shape, with the eardrum at the foot of the L. That means the aid must fit deeper inside to help the dog hear—and it's hard to explain to your dog why you're sticking something inside his ear. Also, the ear itself must otherwise be healthy with no infections. Sticking an aid inside the canal interferes with air circulation and can cause even more infections, says Arvle E. Marshall, DVM, an associate professor in the department of anatomy at Auburn University.

Blanche L. Blackington, a clinical audiologist in San Diego, has partnered with two veterinarians and a hearing-aid engineer to design aids for dogs. The aids have been successfully tested in two dogs—a Boston Terrier and a Lhasa Apso. A return of hearing helps the dog become more active and social, says Blackington.

Dr. Marshall worked on a similar canine hearing-aid project several years ago, but was not successful in getting the dogs to tolerate wearing the aids. "We ended up putting the hearing aid on the collar, and feeding the sound in with a plastic tube," says Dr. Marshall. The end of the tube was

---

COMFORT ZONE

- Getting the attention of a deaf dog can be done by stamping your foot, or by tossing a soft stuffed toy or beanbag into their line of sight. A flashlight may work well at night.
- Remote-control vibrating collars may help. The dog learns to respond to the vibration in the same way he would a voice command. A commercial Vibration Training Collar costs about $115 from Drs. Foster and Smith pet supply.
- Instructions to make a homemade vibrating collar using a Radio Shack remote control car are available on Dr. Strain's Web site at: www.lsu.edu/deafness/deaf.htm

---

held in the ear canal with a foam plug, and had almost no weight to bother the dog. "That was a practical solution," he says.

The owner must be able to train the dog to wear the hearing aid, or you're wasting your time and money. Human hearing aids may cost as much as $1000 to $3000. Some people in the program, though, were delighted to spend $300 on the canine hearing aids and had the time and dedication to make it work, says Dr. Marshall. He says these were the owners who wanted their dog to be happy during the last years of his life.

"We designed a training program that was patterned after training a two-year-old child to wear one," says Dr. Marshall. "It's a reward deal. He leaves it in, he gets his treat." It usually required two to three weeks to train the dog to accept the aid.

Golden Moments: Tazzy's Reawakening

When Carol Kjellsen of Cumming, Georgia, adopted Tazzy, the Shetland Sheepdog/Yorkshire Terrier mix pup was five weeks old and weighed less than twelve ounces. "She looked like a Tasmanian devil!" says Carol. The orphan had no fur, couldn't stand on her own, and wasn't able to nurse properly because her Yorkie mom had died shortly after giving birth.

In the beginning, she was so tiny nobody was sure the pup would survive. For their first month together, Tazzy lived in a little fleece sack Carol carried around in her pocket. Today, Tazzy is fourteen years old, seventeen inches tall, and weighs seventeen pounds. After more than a decade together, the dog and her surrogate "mom" remain closer than ever.

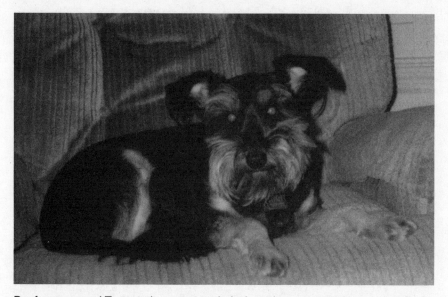

Deafness caused Tazzy to become startled when she was petted unexpectedly. An innovative solution returned her hearing—and reconnected her to life. *(Photo Credit: Carole Kjellsen)*

That's why two years ago, Carol immediately noticed something wasn't quite right. Tazzy wasn't barking as much as usual. "Shelties bark a lot, and she always barked at every noise," says Carol. But Tazzy started sleeping through the doorbell. Then even the sound of the garage door wouldn't rouse her. Touching the dog to wake her up made Tazzy nearly jump out of her skin. Carol knew the hearing loss was impacting her dog's quality of life.

"We travel with our three dogs a lot, and that was fine when she could hear me," says Carol. If the dogs saw and chased something, they were trained to come when called. "When Tazzy's hearing went, that became a problem."

Cataract surgery had saved the eyesight of her cousin's dog, and Carol wondered if hearing aids were also possible. "Everybody thought I was crazy," she says, but she asked her veterinarian anyway.

"Ms. Kjellsen is a very special client," says Dr. Mike McLaughlin of Animal Medical Center in Cumming. "Somebody who considers putting a hearing aid in a dog is up there at the top of the list!" Dr. McLaughlin remembered that while he was in school at Auburn, Dr. Arvle Marshall conducted a research study putting hearing aids in dogs. He called and asked if a hearing aid might help Tazzy.

The first step was to determine if she was deaf or hard of hearing. A test called the brain stem auditory evoked response (BAER test) conducted at Auburn would cost about $500. Another option worked just as well in this situation, though, and cost nothing. Dr. McLaughlin told Carol to wait until Tazzy was awake, make sure the dog couldn't see her, and then whistle. "If you whistle and the ears twitch, the dog can hear to some capacity and is a candidate for a hearing aid," says Dr. McLaughlin. The ear-twitch reflex does not work if the dog is deaf.

Tazzy's ear twitched. She was hard of hearing, and therefore a candidate for an aid.

The next step was training her to accept wearing the foam earplug, says Carol. She was told this training typically took a couple of weeks, and that some dogs never accepted the sensation. But because of their special relationship, Carol never had any doubt that Tazzy would trust her and accept the earplug. "I showed her the earplug, held her really close, and put it in," says Carol. Tazzy wore it for two minutes the first time. When she shook her head, Carol gave her a break and took it out. The next time, Tazzy wore it for fifteen minutes before asking for a break. "The third time she left it in for two hours. And the fourth time, Tazzy left it in for six hours. So I called Mike and said wearing the aid wouldn't be a problem."

The final step was putting together the hearing-aid system for Tazzy. The original Auburn research project was long finished, and no canine hearing aids were left. Recycling a human hearing aid was the best and least expensive option. Carol's father-in-law donated one of his old hearing aids to the project.

The hearing aid was attached to Tazzy's collar with Velcro. Then a small piece of IV tubing connected the hearing aid to the foam earplug, and the foam plug was inserted into Tazzy's ear. "Then I put the batteries in, and Tazzy immediately reacted!" says Carol. "It was very obvious she was hearing. She'd go outside and her little head would go up. The barking started again and I thought, 'Oh, gee, I forgot that!' "

Suddenly Tazzy could hear crickets and birds—and other dogs again. Patti the Pekingese rattles the walls with her snores, says Carol, and it used to disturb Tazzy so much she'd bark to be rescued. "One of the first things I noticed was Tazzy looking at Patti snoring as if to say, 'Why am I hearing this again?' "

There are times when the dog prefers not to hear everything. She's learned to tell Carol when the batteries go dead, or if the hearing aid whistles with feedback—Tazzy simply paws out the aid. "Her ears get sore if she wears it every single day, so we just put it in when we need to, such as when we travel," says Carol. The hearing aid has reawakened the close connection the pair share, and opened the world back up for Tazzy.

Dental Disease

Eighty percent of dogs develop periodontal disease by age three. Smaller dogs have the greatest risk because of their large teeth crowding their small jaws.

"In all animals, the most common disease of any in the pet population is periodontal disease," says Bill Gengler, DVM. "The longer they are on the planet, the more at risk they are, If you looked at the older patient, the incidence would rise noticeably," he says.

Dogs don't chew their food very much, and so won't benefit from the scrubbing or detergent action the way people do. Wet food tends to stick to the teeth more than dry food, which means dry food may help prevent tooth deposits. But recent studies have not found a significant benefit in feeding dogs dry food versus semimoist or wet food. On average, dry food probably improves dental hygiene by about 10 percent, say veterinary dentists. The effect of hard food on dental health also varies according to the individual animal.

Periodontal disease is a group of disorders that affect the teeth, oral bones, and the gums. Just like people, dogs are prone to bacterial grown on the tooth surface that creates plaque and bad breath. When plaque isn't removed through normal chewing or brushing of the dog's teeth, it mineralizes into tartar that forms hard yellow or brown deposits. The bacteria releases enzymes that attack the dog's gums and cause gingivitis (inflammation of the gums), gum recession, loose or lost teeth, and pain.

SENIOR SYMPTOMS

Owners often neglect the dog's teeth because they don't notice he's having any problems. "Usually in the early stages, anyway, animals will eat through the pain because the self-preservation instinct is so strong," says Dr. Gengler. What you will see includes:

- Redness of the gums
- Receding gum line
- Strong offensive odor
- Blood on the toothbrush or chew toys
- Broken teeth
- Loose teeth
- Missing teeth

Less frequently, dogs get cavities. But mouth infections and gum or tooth disease impact the overall health of your dog because bacteria can get into their bloodstream and damage organs in other areas of the body.

Teeth can also be damaged during a lifetime of wear, causing pain and impacting behavior. Dogs use their mouths and teeth not only like a hand to hold and pick up objects; they also indulge in a great deal of recreational chewing. Poorly chosen chew objects, such as a chain-link fence, stones, or wood, can wear down or even break teeth.

"People think that because an animal has been eating well, that a broken tooth doesn't bother them," says Dr. Gengler, but that's not the case. Painful teeth can affect the dog's behavior in many ways. Typically, though, behavior changes are so gradual that owners don't attribute them to a painful mouth. "Just like us, a broken tooth doesn't ache all the time," says Dr. Gengler. When there's a flare-up the dog may simply retreat and hide under the bed, or decline to play.

Usually, dogs eat through the pain, until they reach the later stages of dental disease when their teeth become loose. Dr. Gengler says, "When we finally treat the tooth the owners call me back and say, 'Wow—my dog is doing what he did five or six years ago! And I thought he was slowing down because of age.'"

TREATMENT

"You can't have them just jump into the dental chair. They won't say 'Ah.' Everything has to be done under anesthetic," says Steven E. Holmstrom, DVM.

COMFORT ZONE

A variety of products are available to help with plaque control.

- Chlorhexidine and zinc ascorbate will kill the bacteria that cause periodontal disease. Commercial products are available in topical gels, rinses, and chew toys, and help prevent and treat dental disease.
- Rawhide chews have a positive benefit on dental health.
- Dental hygiene chew toys, such as Hercules Bones are available at most pet product outlets and come in three sizes: regular (dogs under thirty pounds), Wolf (thirty to sixty pounds), and Souper (over sixty pounds). They are covered with raised dental tips and enhanced with chicken flavor. Such chew toys have been found to decrease calculus, plaque, and the incidence and severity of gingivitis in dogs after three or four weeks.
- Avoid offering very hard chew toys. Periodontal disease can weaken teeth and predispose dogs to pathological fractures that may result simply from chewing a hard object, like an ice cube, cow hoof, or hard nylon bone.
- A natural commercial product called Greenies, available at Drs. Foster and Smith and other pet supply outlets, are also a big hit with dogs. Greenies are treats made from human food–grade ingredients and include natural chlorophyll for fresh breath.
- Fresh carrots and apple slices also provide dental benefits, and many dogs enjoy chewing and eating crunchy vegetables and fruit.

The first step is to check the dog for any potential anesthetic risk. "This is particularly important in geriatric pets," says Dr. Holmstrom, because they have other health conditions that make them more sensitive. Screening tests evaluate the blood chemistry, electrolytes, liver and kidney function, blood cells and platelet status, urinalysis, or even the heart using tests such as electrocardiograms (ECG or EKG).

A preanesthetic evaluation allows the veterinarian to make sure the anesthetic is safe—to allow for a heart condition, for example. "It oftentimes will

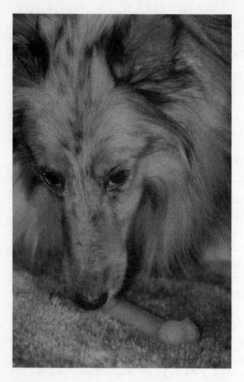

Choose from a wide range of canine dental chew products for your dog. *(Photo Credit: Amy D. Shojai)*

identify subclinical disease that maybe has nothing to do with dentistry," says Dr. Gengler. That makes the owner aware that something else is going on—say, kidney failure—that calls for a change of diet that can make that animal a lot more comfortable and live longer.

Most veterinarians are able to offer routine dental care, such as cleaning and extractions, when necessary. Veterinary dentists have the benefit of additional training and more specialized equipment. Root canals, crowns, and orthodontia for medical reasons are quite common. Teeth that are misaligned may damage the dog's mouth as he chews, and need to be realigned to prevent serious injury. Those veterinary dentists practicing at specialty practices or teaching hospitals have the added advantage of having access to veterinary anesthesiologists.

Typically, once the dog is cleared for dentistry, an anesthetic such as isofluorine or sebofluorine is administered. In older patients, Dr. Holmstrom says fluids are also helpful to counteract potential hypotension (low blood pressure) that may result from the anesthetic.

"The next step is evaluating all the teeth with a periodontal probe," says Dr. Holmstrom. "Dental X rays are extremely beneficial to detect lesions below the gum line, and getting an idea of bone loss." Then tartar is scaled away. If necessary, teeth are pulled. Many times, tartar is all that's holding bad teeth in place, and once that's gone, they almost fall out on their own.

Once there's active periodontal disease, more than one treatment usually is required. Antibiotics often are prescribed afterward to fight infection and counteract new problems that may develop from the open wounds (pockets) associated with the disease.

Dogs usually do quite well with tooth loss, though. Dr. Holmstrom says it's best to keep the canines (fang teeth) and carnassial teeth (big molars) that do most of the chewing. "The lower canine teeth act as a guide for the tongue, and the upper ones keep the lip away from the gum tissue," he says. Without these teeth, the dog may have trouble keeping his tongue in his mouth.

BOTTOM LINE

Cost for professional dental care for dogs varies, but the anesthetic, antibiotics, and cleaning combined usually runs about $150.

PREVENTION

Every dog is different, and some have more problems with tartar than others. In young dogs, once-a-year teeth cleaning at the vet might be adequate. "But as the animal ages, chances are they may need more care professionally," says Dr. Gengler. Dogs such as Yorkshire Terriers that are highly prone to dental disease may need attention two to four times a year, especially if owners aren't able to provide home dental care. "Once the animal loses its natural defense mechanism and pockets are formed and bone is lost, that is not regained. It doesn't heal naturally," says Dr. Gengler. "That animal is going to be a much higher-maintenance animal."

The best way to deal with canine dental disease is to brush your dog's teeth every day. Even once or twice a week is better than never. Start slowly, find a toothpaste flavor your dog likes, and use it like a treat, suggests Dr. Holmstrom. "Avoid human toothpaste. They often don't like the flavor, and there are detergents in it that shouldn't be swallowed," he says. Dogs aren't able to spit, and the foaming action is unpleasant and can upset their stomachs.

FEEDING FOR HEALTH

Although these diets can help with dental care, be sure the diet itself is appropriate for your dog's total health requirements. The need for a therapeutic kidney diet may override dental concerns, for example.

- Eukanuba Dental Defense System (added to all adult Eukanuba foods)
- Hill's Science Diet Oral Care
- Hill's Prescription Diet Canine t/d (available only from veterinarian)
- Nutro Natural Choice Dental Care

Poultry- and beef-flavored pet toothpastes are commercially available and are made for animals to swallow. These pastes may include the enzymes glucose oxidase and lactoperoxidase, which have antimicrobial activity and aid in plaque control.

AGE-DEFYING TIPS

Keeping the dog's teeth clean and healthy throughout his life provides a positive impact on his total health, improves quality of life as he ages, and may add to longevity. In addition to brushing your dog's teeth, a dental diet may help prevent dental disease.

- Look for sodium hexametaphosphate (sodium HMP) listed in the food. This helps to prevent plaque from attaching to the tooth surface. More and more "regular" pet diets contain sodium HMP as a part of the formula. Some diets with dental claims include polyphosphate crystals to help prevent the mineralization of plaque into calculus.
- Some diets offer a scrubbing action to clean the tooth as the dog chews by way of unique fibers in the food.
- Look for the "Veterinary Oral Health Council (VOHC) Seal of Acceptance." That means the product has passed a rigorous and objective review of effectiveness from representatives from the fields of veterinary dentistry and dental science along with representatives of the American Dental Association, American Veterinary Medical Association, and American Animal Hospital Association.

Dog toothbrushes are also available, or choose a preschool size human toothbrush with the softest bristles. "Put the paste on the brush, let them lick the brush three or four times a day without making any effort to brush the teeth for several weeks, until the pet's coming to you to beg for treat time," says Dr. Holmstrom. Gradually progress to handling the dog's mouth until he's more comfortable. Once the dog is completely comfortable with the idea, he suggests putting a dog toy in his mouth to prop it open, put your hand around his muzzle to hold him steady and keep the toy in place, then brush the teeth.

Diabetes Mellitus

Diabetes is a general term that refers to several disorders that share similar symptoms but have different causes. Diabetes insipidus typically affects puppies or young-adult dogs, and results from a lack of the hormone vasopressin (ADH) that controls water resorption in the kidneys. Diabetes mellitus is much more common, and most dogs are middle-aged or older when they develop symptoms.

Diabetes mellitus is a metabolic disorder in which insulin is not produced by the pancreas in sufficient quantities (Type I, insulin dependent), or the body is unable to use the insulin that's present (Type II, noninsulin dependent). Insulin is a hormone that makes possible the movement of glucose (sugar) from the blood into the cells of the body, where it is used for energy. Although the dog's body may be able to process food into glucose, the diabetic animal is unable to use this energy and slowly starves.

The unused glucose in the bloodstream spills into the urine, and this sugary liquid acts to pull even more water out of the body in a process called osmotic diuresis. That makes the dog thirsty, so she drinks more, which increases her need to urinate. Often the first sign an owner notices is a break in housetraining, when the dog is unable to "hold it" to get outside in time. Symptoms point to the disease, and diagnosis is confirmed by testing the blood and urine.

A large percentage of body fat tends to suppress insulin function, which is why a large percentage of diabetic dogs are also overweight. "Obesity

definitely doubles, triples, or quadruples your risk for diabetes," says Dottie LaFlamme, DVM. Damage to the pancreas, such as chronic pancreatitis, also can cause the disease.

SENIOR SYMPTOMS

Various signs of diabetes can be similar to symptoms of other serious
illnesses, such as kidney disease or age-related urinary incontinence.

- Increased thirst
- Increased urination
- Sticky, "sugary" urine
- Break in housetraining
- Increased appetite
- Weight loss
- Cataracts and blindness
- Bad breath that smells sweetish, like nail polish

About one in two hundred dogs develops diabetes. Females are affected
twice as often as male dogs. Breeds most commonly affected include
Samoyeds, Miniature Schnauzers, Miniature/Toy Poodles, and Pugs. "It's
an old-animal diagnosis," says Richard Nelson, DVM. "The average age of
diagnosis is ten years for dogs," he says, noting that with proper treatment,
most live with a good quality of life for another three years after diagnosis
until they're thirteen or fourteen years of age.

TREATMENT

Dr. Nelson says it's important to remember that diabetes in dogs is not
the same as diabetes in people. "In people diabetes causes a lot of chronic
complications that have a negative impact on survival time," says Dr. Nelson, so very rigid control of the disease is necessary to prevent complications that may happen forty years from now. But dogs don't live that long,
he says, so they don't have to worry about such complications.

"We're trying to keep them active and reasonably healthy, happy, stable
body weight, control accidents in the house, reasonable water intake, inter-
active with family members—that's really our goal. It's a quality-of-life
issue," says Dr. Nelson.

FEEDING FOR HEALTH

A high-fiber diet not only helps reduce overweight, but also helps regulate the rate at which food is digested and glucose released into the dog's system. A number of diets may be appropriate, including:

- Eukanuba Veterinary Diets, Nutritional Weight Maintenance Formula, Glucose-Control/Canine
- Eukanuba Veterinary Diets, Nutritional Weight Maintenance Formula, Senior Plus/Canine
- Eukanuba Veterinary Diets, Nutritional Weight Loss Formula, Restricted-Calorie/Canine
- IVD Select Care Canine Hifactor Formula
- IVD Select Care Canine Mature
- Nutro Max Weight Control Formula
- Precise Light Formula for Less Active or Overweight Dogs
- Purina Veterinary Diets, DCO Diabetes Colitis Formula
- Waltham Canine Glucomodulation Control Diet

A small percentage of Type II dogs may benefit from oral diabetic medication called glipizide (Glucotrol) that boosts the production of insulin in the pancreas. A new supplement on the market, S-Adenosylmethionine (SAMe) is a kind of nutraceutical antioxidant, which may be helpful in diabetic dogs that develop liver complications. Supplementation with S-Adenosylmethionine (Denosyl SD4) has been demonstrated to improve liver function in these pets.

Dr. Nelson says 99.9 percent of diabetic dogs require insulin injections, usually twice a day. Various types of insulin are available, and different ones may work better for individual dogs. "Right now the insulins of choice for me in the dog are humulin, lente, or recombinant human lente," says Dr. Nelson. The amount of insulin needed depends on the dog's size, activity level, and metabolism, among other factors, and it may take time to regulate the patient.

Once the veterinarian has determined the dosage, most owners become proficient in giving insulin injections. They may also use urine test strips to help monitor glucose levels in the dog's urine, in order to adjust the dose or frequency if necessary. How much the dog eats or exercises influences glucose levels. Maintaining a regular routine is important. Too much insulin or too little can have devastating consequences.

Diabetic coma may result if the dog gets the wrong amount, if she doesn't eat on schedule, or if she overexercises. The dog loses conscious-

---

AGE-DEFYING TIP

"The single best thing an individual could do in terms of trying to minimize the potential development of diabetes is weight control, and trying to avoid obesity," says Dr. Nelson. "That causes insulin resistance and has been shown to be a definite cause-and-effect factor in dogs and cats both."

---

ness and can't be awakened. This is a life-threatening emergency that requires immediate veterinary help.

Too much insulin can prompt hypoglycemia, also called insulin reaction. The dog acts disoriented or drunk, drools, shakes, acts weak, and may develop a head tilt. Giving her a glucose source such as honey or Karo syrup should reverse these signs in five to fifteen minutes. Without intervention, the condition progresses to convulsions, coma, and death.

"Most diabetic dogs, at least in the early stage, are overweight," says Debbie Davenport, DVM. "Our recommendation would be a moderate-fiber diet that has controlled levels of calories." Reducing the weight with a veterinary-supervised low-calorie, high-fiber diet and moderate exercise is considered a keystone of diabetic treatment. Diets with higher fiber not only help reduce weight, but also take longer for the dog to digest. That helps maintain glucose levels in the bloodstream in a more even pattern.

Usually blood tests are monitored for blood sugar levels, and the amount and frequency of insulin administration is adjusted accordingly. More recently, veterinarians test the blood for levels of fructosamine, a glycan protein. "It's a marker of average blood sugars over a period of two to three weeks, and it's not affected by stress. So it's a little bit more objective information on how well the animal's been regulated," says Dr. Nelson. "If you can keep most of your blood sugar under two hundred throughout the day, dogs are relatively [symptom-free], and they do just fine."

Golden Moments: Heidi Sticks It Out

Tina and Bob Horton of Braceville, Illinois, were not looking for another dog. They had just lost their German Shepherd to cancer, and had their hands full with Crystal, an elderly white rescue Poodle. "Our anniversary was coming up, and we said, 'Let's look at the shelter.' It was just curiosity," says Tina.

Then a sad-looking dog took one look at the pair and began jumping up and down, as though begging, "Take me! Take me!" "I said to my husband, 'This is the one,' " says Tina. Heidi became their anniversary present to each other that year.

It was an even better present for the eight-month-old Greyhound-Doberman mix. The brindle-colored dog had been scheduled for euthanasia because her temperament was so poor. "She had scars all over her legs that they thought were cigarette burns," says Tina. The shelter staff said they'd take her back and return the adoption fee if there was no improvement in her behavior in four weeks.

Tina was determined to give the scared, abused dog the chance for a happy home. "We took her home, and we couldn't touch her. She would spend hours outside in the big fenced yard, then come in, go in the room, and poop. Every day this happened two or three times," she says. Tina was patient, though. "I never raised my hand; she never knew what a slap was. I just trained her with my voice, saying, 'Good girl,' or 'Bad girl.' " It took six weeks for Heidi to learn to trust her new owners and turn the corner.

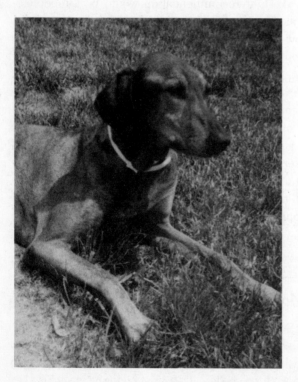

Heidi's symptoms were reversed once she was diagnosed and treated for diabetes. *(Photo Credit: Tina Horton)*

"Heidi became a very happy dog," says Tina. They belonged to a recreation club and would take the big dog back in the woods and fields. There, Heidi could really cut loose. "Oh, gosh, could she run!" says Tina. "She just loved it. There was no stopping her."

When Heidi was eight, the Hortons came home to find a big puddle on the kitchen floor. The next day they found another puddle. They thought Crystal, their sixteen-year-old Poodle, had done it, but they were never able to catch the culprit in the act.

Then Heidi developed a terrible smell, says Tina. A bath and cologne didn't help, so they took her to the veterinarian. Because of her age, he suspected Heidi's accidents were due to age-related urinary incontinence, a common condition of aging spayed female dogs. But an injection of diethylstilbestrol (DES), estrogen replacement therapy that helps some dogs, had no effect. She continued to have accidents, and the smell persisted. She also had begun to lose a lot of weight.

The veterinarian finally diagnosed diabetes. "He gave me a pill to give her once a day, but it didn't help anything," says Tina. By this time Heidi was in terrible shape. The awful smell was due to ketoacidosis, a rather late-stage sign of diabetes when the body begins to break down its own muscles for energy because the diabetes prevents normal metabolism of glucose. When the veterinarian could offer no further hope, he suggested they put Heidi to sleep.

"My husband and I were both heartbroken," says Tina. "My husband said, 'Second opinion. Let's go somewhere else!' " If another veterinarian agreed with the verdict, they'd say good-bye to Heidi and put the sweet dog to sleep.

They took Heidi to the Dwight Veterinary Clinic in Dwight, Illinois. Dr. Louis Cronin examined her.

Heidi had dropped from seventy pounds to forty-three pounds. "She was just skin and bones and horrible to look at, and he didn't know if she was too far gone," says Tina. Dr. Cronin explained there were no guarantees, that her kidneys might be damaged, and that her liver enzymes were high. But insulin injections were Heidi's only hope of survival.

Tina and Bob were willing to try anything to save Heidi's life. "But I had never had a syringe in my hands; I was so scared!" says Tina. "I couldn't do it. And my husband couldn't do it." Each time she tried to give the injection as Dr. Cronin had demonstrated, Heidi jumped. "One time I gave myself a shot; it went right into my finger," says Tina. She returned to the clinic, crying her heart out to Dr. Cronin that she couldn't do it, couldn't give Heidi the shots.

Tina says he wouldn't let her give up. Each morning for a week Tina brought the dog to the office, and was given step-by-step hands-on training on how to pick her skin up, insert the needle, and give the lifesaving insulin. "He'd say, 'You can do it, you *can* do it, you *love* her—you can do it!' " And finally it sank in with me. From one day to the next, I could do it," says Tina.

The first days and weeks were terrible, and Dr. Cronin seemed just as concerned about Heidi as Bob and Tina were. He often called to see how "our Heidi" was doing, says Tina. "He gave me his home phone number in case anything happened, said I should call even at one o'clock in the morning and he'd meet me at the office. I had to do that twice."

The insulin injections were increased to twice a day. Every time the dog got a shot she got a special treat. "She wanted the treat so bad that she learned to tell me that it's time for the shot," says Tina. "She's good; she never moves."

Heidi was beginning to make a comeback, but she desperately needed to regain the lost weight. For three weeks the Hortons took her every day to the drive-in because she liked the hamburgers there. "Then we changed to tunafish sandwiches with hardboiled eggs and she would eat those. She was getting really spoiled." Finally, after Heidi had regained the first ten pounds of what had been lost, she went back to eating dog food.

Five years later, at age thirteen, Heidi has her weight back and is doing very well. "Dr. Cronin is just a fantastic vet," says Tina. "If it wasn't for him, Heidi wouldn't be around. Our animals are family members. Our kids are all gone; they live all around the United States—our pets are our kids now. And they love us back."

NURSE ALERT!

Should your dog be diagnosed with diabetes, at-home insulin shots will be required from once to several times a day.

Dry Eye

Dry eye is a loss of tear production. It's usually seen as a genetic condition in certain breeds of dog, such as Cocker Spaniels, Shih Tzus, and Bulldogs, but any dog as he gets older can experience a loss of tearing. That can allow the cornea to get drier and more likely to become irritated. Chronic inflammation of the conjunctiva, called conjunctivitis, can develop, and dogs suffering from dry eye become more prone to eye infections.

SENIOR SYMPTOMS

Dry eye may not be painful initially, but it can lead to other problems that cause pain. Consequently, the symptoms may mimic other eye problems.

- Sleepy crusts or morning "stuff"
- An accumulation of mucus
- Increased blinking or squinting

TREATMENT

In most cases, home treatment is all that's needed. Owners should keep the dog's hair out of his eyes, to help prevent abrasions or contamination. Also keep the eyes clean with an eyewash and cotton balls, and wipe away excess mucus.

If further problems develop, such as increased crusts, squinting, or pawing/rubbing at the eye, a veterinary exam will be required. "The veterinarian can check their tear production and if it's low they can supplement it with artificial tears," says Harriet Davidson, DVM.

A drug called cyclosporine (Optimmune) can increase the animal's own natural tear production. Dr. Davidson adds, "This is a 0.2 concentration, a tiny amount, but it works wonderfully."

NURSE ALERT!

Dogs with longish fur that falls over their eyes benefit from having it trimmed or tied back, and always kept clean. It's tricky cutting hair close to the eyes, so unless your dog is very laid-back, ask your veterinarian to demonstrate at least the first time. Other eye care you'll need to perform:

- Wipe away "sleepy crusts." Soak a cotton ball with warm water or contact lens saline solution, hold against dried secretions until they soften, and clean away.
- Artificial Tears eye drops—the same ones you use are fine.
- Optimmune ointment, or other prescribed eye medicine.

Glaucoma

Glaucoma is an extremely painful disease in which pressure increases inside the eyeball, and pushes the internal structures out of position. It can cause sudden blindness in as little as twenty-four hours, or can develop over weeks to months. Without treatment, the dog will go blind.

A fluid called aqueous humor fills the front part of the eyeball and keeps the internal structures in the proper places. In a normal eye, the level of the liquid remains constant as the same amount that's produced is drained away. This works in a similar fashion to a faucet in a sink, where the water drains away as fast as it pours in. Glaucoma develops if not enough fluid is drained away, and the eyeball swells with the excess pressure.

Secondary glaucoma develops as a result of disease or injury that interferes with this natural flow of fluid. "Dogs can certainly develop glaucoma as a result of untreated cataracts," says Paul A. Gerding, Jr., DVM. Primary disease, though, develops spontaneously and is thought to be heritable in Beagles. It also frequently affects Cocker Spaniels, Basset Hounds, and Siberian Huskies or other Arctic Circle breeds. "Uveitis [inflammation of the eye] can lead to glaucoma," says Harriet Davidson, DVM. "The animal will tend to keep its head guarded, keep that eye away from you, and won't want you to touch it."

An instrument such as a Schiotz tonometer or TonoPen measures the pressure inside the eyeball to diagnose the condition. The tonometer is gently balanced on the dog's cornea (after drops numb the area), and a scale on the instrument indicates the pressure. The TonoPen is much smaller and contains a computer microchip that registers a reading when it's merely tapped on the surface of the eye.

SENIOR SYMPTOMS

Glaucoma is a progressive disease that develops relatively slowly in people, but is very aggressive in dogs and can lead to blindness. The primary symptom is excruciating pain. Signs to watch for include:

- Excessive tearing
- Cloudy or bloodshot eye
- Squinting or pawing at the painful eye
- Tipping head to relieve pressure from the aggravated side
- Keeping eyelid closed, or pulling away from touch
- Dilated and unresponsive pupil
- Enlarged eyeball

NURSE ALERT!

- Once glaucoma is diagnosed, your dog will require eyedrops to be administered several times a day, perhaps for the rest of his life.
- Should he require surgery to remove the eyeball, watching the area and keeping the socket clean with warm water on a cotton ball will be important to guard against infection. You may also need to apply ointment to the surgery site until it's fully healed.
- A collar restraint may be necessary to prevent your dog from pawing at and damaging his sore eye. Dogs may have trouble eating while wearing an E-collar, so remove it during meals and supervise his activity.

TREATMENT

"Glaucoma is an emergency. You need to have an animal evaluated by the veterinarian and treated immediately," says Dr. Davidson. It takes only a few days for permanent damage to occur.

The condition is treated very aggressively. Eyedrops such as Xalatan and latanoprost are particularly helpful for dogs. The drops help to relieve the pain, contract the pupil, and reduce the inflammation. If medication fails to control the condition, surgery may be necessary.

When glaucoma affects one eye as a primary cause—not from an injury—it often eventually develops in the other eye as well. "If we're able to catch one eye, we stand a good chance of delaying the onset in the other one with preventive treatment," says Dr. Gerding. Dogs typically stop responding to this long-term medical care, though, and usually both eyes will be affected by glaucoma.

Veterinary ophthalmologists offer a couple of different surgical options. Tiny shunts may be implanted to help control the pressure by draining away excess fluid. Cryosurgery to freeze the fluid-producing cells in the ciliary epithelium also is an option. One of the most recent and successful innovations uses an ophthalmic-size laser to perform a procedure called laser ciliary body ablation. The laser selectively destroys fluid-producing tissues in the eye, and so reduces fluid production, says Dr. Gerding.

When the disease has progressed to where the pupil no longer responds to light, the dog has lost vision in that eye. If medication can't control the pain, then several surgical options are available. The most common procedure involves a scleral prosthesis—a silicon ball—that's placed inside the damaged eyeball after the painful internal structures have been removed. This is also a good cosmetic procedure, in which the dog keeps his eye, and the eyeball will still move, but he'll have no vision.

Another possibility is to remove the eyeball altogether, in a procedure called enucleation. If enucleation is performed, a prosthetic implant may be placed, or sometimes the socket is left empty, and the eyelid is sewn shut.

Dogs that have lost the vision in one or both eyes tend to do extremely well and adjust quickly. Removing the pain often returns the dog to a higher activity level because she feels so much better.

BOTTOM LINE

- Costs to treat glaucoma vary from $300 to $1000, depending on the type and severity of glaucoma and the size of the dog.
- Cost to implant the prosthetic implant generally runs about $600 per eye.

Heart Disease

Heart failure results when the damaged muscle is no longer able to move blood properly throughout the body. Heart disease occurs in about 11 percent of all dogs. Dogs may be born with congenital heart problems such as patent ductus arteriosus (PDA), which requires surgery to fix. Certain breeds of dogs, such as Boxers, Cocker Spaniels, and Dobermans, are more prone to dilated cardiomyopathy, in which the heart muscle enlarges and cannot adequately contract to pump blood. Dilated cardiomyopathy is not an old-dog problem, though, and dogs are typically diagnosed with it at three to five years of age.

Many pets have heart disease, but can often remain symptom-free for many years. Just because the pet has a heart problem doesn't mean it will affect his well-being or life span. Heart disease becomes life-threatening in only one of three ways: cardiac arrhythmia (irregular heartbeat), thromboembolic disease (blood clot or stroke), or congestive heart failure.

Most heart problems affect dogs during their senior years, says Rhonda Schulman, DVM. Heart disease may develop due to cancer, parasites such as heartworms, or damage from infectious diseases. For example, the bacterium from periodontal disease contributes to heart problems in older dogs. Valvular heart disease affects about one-third of all dogs over the age of twelve. The heart valves simply begin to wear out, and leak blood backward instead of pumping it all forward. This puts extra strain on the heart muscle.

Heart disease has a cascading effect on the whole body, and can compromise other organs such as the kidneys, liver, and lungs. When the left side of the heart fails, fluid collects in the lungs (pulmonary edema) and makes it hard to breathe. "Breathing problems and coughing can be a distinct and most significant clue, but they tend to be later findings," says Dr. Schulman.

SENIOR SYMPTOMS

There are several different kinds of heart disease, and symptoms vary from type to type. They include:

- Tires easily
- Weakness
- Bluish tinge to the skin from lack of oxygen
- Swollen abdomen or legs
- Coughing, especially at night
- Labored breathing
- Loss of appetite
- Sitting with "elbows" outward and/or neck extended to aid breathing

---

When the right side of the heart fails, fluid collects and swells the abdomen (ascites), accumulates beneath the skin (edema—the legs may swell), and/or fills the chest cavity (pleural effusion). Fluids collect when the body tries to compensate for reduced heart efficiency. Sodium and fluid are retained to increase blood volume, and blood vessels are constricted to increase blood pressure. Dogs suffering from congestive heart failure will have a heart murmur. Many times, right heart failure develops as a result of the strain from existing left heart failure.

DIAGNOSIS

"A lot of times we'll hear something abnormal when we scope them," says Dr. Schulman. Simply listening with a stethoscope may detect a murmur or excessive fluid in the lungs, she says. "Radiographs [X rays] of the thorax will typically show an enlarged heart, and you might see changes in the lungs consistent with fluid." Most veterinarians have X-ray machines in their offices and will be able to make a general diagnosis.

An echocardiogram, or ultrasound of the heart, is the ideal way to diagnose heart disease. That requires specialized equipment that general-practice veterinarians usually don't have. Typically dogs will be referred to a veterinary cardiologist or internist. The echocardiogram tells the veterinarian a great deal, says Sheila McCullough, DVM, including how strongly the heart is able to contract, and if there are any leaky valves. "It gives you a better idea of the heart chamber size, the thickness or thinness of the walls." Thorough testing helps determine which medications will work best for the dog. "We often do re-echoes after they've been put on the medication to see if they're actually improving," she says.

BOTTOM LINE

Cost for diagnostic tests vary in different parts of the country, and the treatment depends on the dog's size and specific requirements. Usually the medication itself is quite reasonable once the problem is diagnosed.

- Echocardiogram costs in the $300 range
- X rays typically start at around $50 to $75 and go up from there
- Open-heart surgeries can cost up to $6000

TREATMENT

The newest frontier in valvular heart disease treatment is open-heart surgery to either repair the native valve or replace it with an artificial valve. These cutting-edge procedures are available only at a handful of veterinary schools, such as Colorado State and University of Pennsylvania, and are considered experimental, risky, and very expensive.

More commonly, medical management is the treatment of choice. "Very few heart diseases are corrected with surgery, so it's normally something that's not cured but controlled," says Dr. Schulman.

Dogs with acquired valvular heart disease can often be helped with drugs that improve the heart's performance and reduce fluid accumulation. Digitalis or related medicines such as Cardoxin or Lanoxin help improve heart muscle performance. Calcium channel blockers such as diltiazem, or beta blockers such as propranolol may help.

A diuretic drug such as Lasix (furosemide) forces the kidneys to eliminate excess salt and water. Diuretics cause the dog to drink more water and urinate more frequently, so extra bathroom stops will be necessary until the body adjusts to the medicine. ACE inhibitors, such as enalapril (Enacard), benazepril (Fortekor), and lisinopril, are vasodilator drugs that ease the workload on the heart by opening up the arteries.

FEEDING FOR HEALTH

Your veterinarian may suggest a number of therapeutic diets designed to help dogs with heart disease, including:

- Hill's Prescription Diet Canine h/d
- IVD Selected Care Canine Modified Formula
- Purina Veterinary Diets, CV Cardiovascular Formula
- Waltham Canine Veterinary Diet Early Cardiac Support

Specially designed therapeutic diets that are low in sodium help the dog compensate for the potassium, chloride, and magnesium lost due to increased fluid excretion, and help them avoid fluid retention. A variety of brands are available, and it's important to choose one that will both be good for the dog, and that he'll readily eat. It may be helpful to feed several small meals to help stimulate the appetite and reduce gastrointestinal upset.

Treatment for congestive heart failure does not correct the problem; it only seeks to alleviate the worst symptoms. Most, though not all, patients who experience congestive heart failure survive as long as they receive treatment promptly, but the long-term outcome for patients is guarded. The goal is to keep the dog comfortable, and maintain a good quality of life despite heart problems.

Golden Moments: Saving Zoë

The news reports described the heartbreaking scene: several breeds of dogs, from puppy to adult, were left without food or water for many weeks when their elderly owner was hospitalized. Of the seventy to eighty dogs, about a dozen were already dead or beyond help when animal control stepped into the situation. "They found these dogs in kennels and in holes in the ground," says Pam Gauthier of Sherman, Texas. Many of the terriers had created their own dirty burrows for shelter and survived by drinking rainwater. The city shelter impounded the surviving dogs, but could house them for only a few days before their resources were exhausted—after that, the dogs would be destroyed.

Pam and her daughter Becky were among several families who responded to the news reports and offered new homes for the neglected dogs. "We were looking at another dog, then found out about Zoë," says Pam. They wanted an older dog that would get along with their other pets, and knew an older dog would be less rambunctious and sedate. "The shelter staff had to make sure Zoë was kenneled with another dog, or she'd climb out. She didn't want to be by herself," says Pam. Zoë had lived with so many other dogs for so long, being kenneled alone was an emotional shock.

The staff had already bathed the Wirehaired Fox Terrier twice, but Zoë was still matted, smelly, and nasty. Information on the dog was sketchy, but Zoë was estimated to be nine to eleven years old. "She was real thin, but friendly as all get out, just a sweetheart," says Pam. Zoë was bathed one more time before Pam took her home. Under the dirt there was an apricot-white-and-black teddy bear of a dog.

Because Zoë had not been handled much during her previous life, she was timid about being held. "Her entire body would stiffen," says Pam. But Zoë got along great with Becky's Dachshund and Pam's Poodle. Zoë quickly claimed a four-inch-deep box as her new bed, and enjoyed curling up inside to sleep next to Pam's bed each night. She also discovered the joys of snuggling on a blanket on the couch. In a very short time, Zoë felt like one of the family.

The adoption fee included a veterinary examination by a participating local clinic. Considering the years of neglect, the dog had managed to keep herself relatively healthy, but for one serious thing: the veterinarian said Zoë had heartworms.

Heartworms are a parasite that is carried by mosquitoes. Infected mosquitoes transmit the baby worms (microfilariae) to the dog when they take a blood meal. These immature worms migrate in the dog's body, and eventually find the heart and pulmonary arteries, where they mature. A heart filled with these parasites can't work efficiently and eventually develops heart disease and congestive heart failure.

Very effective and inexpensive medications—often given once a month as a chewable pill—prevent this infection. But Zoë had never received the benefit of proper veterinary care or preventive heartworm medicines. Once a dog is infected with heartworms, the treatment to cure the problem is not only expensive; it can be dangerous—and may not completely reverse the heart damage.

"It was about $300 minimum to do the blood work, X rays, pretreatment and posttreatment stuff," says Pam. The various tests would determine what stage of the disease Zoë was in, which would help determine the best way to treat her.

The typical treatment for heartworm disease involves injecting the dog with an arseniclike drug to kill the worms. This may be given over a period of two days, or sometimes over the period of two months, which may be less stressful for very ill dogs. In any treatment, complications may develop when the dead worms break apart and move into the bloodstream. If they block the flow of blood and cause a clot—an embolism—the dog could die. A third treatment option that uses the heartworm preventative for eighteen months may work with young, otherwise healthy dogs, but the veterinarian told Pam that given Zoë's age, the eighteen-month plan probably would kill her.

Pam struggled with the decision whether or not to treat Zoë. "If I take her for heartworm treatment, I could be condemning her to death. But she's already got the heartworms so she's already condemned to death," says Pam. "We're not rich people—we opted not to do the blood work. But I wanted as many opinions as I could get."

She had the dog examined by another veterinarian, and had X rays done to better judge the dog's condition. Zoë's heart was enlarged, and she had fluid in her belly (ascites) as a result of the heart failure. Based on the X rays, the veterinarian agreed that the eighteen-month and the two-day treatments were risky, but said Zoë probably could survive the two-month heartworm treatment plan. "The veterinarian also said to give her baby aspirin to prevent blood clots," says Pam. Zoë was to take one baby aspirin each day for three weeks before and three weeks after the treatment.

Pam took the dog to one more veterinarian—Dr. Freda Wells of Bryan County Animal Hospital—and provided the doctor with the X-ray results and information she had gathered. "Doc Freda offered to do the treatment for about $60," says Pam. "She said to bring Zoë home and fatten her up for about a month first."

Zoë loves food, so fattening her up wasn't a problem. If food wasn't in her bowl, she scrounged until she found some. "I came home one day and

---

NURSING ALERT!

Heart medications are usually administered in pill form, but sometimes they come as liquids. You'll need to administer heart medicine for the rest of the dog's life.

- If the dog is allowed to eat other food, you can "hide" the pill in a tiny bit of low-fat cream cheese, peanut butter, or cheese.
- If a therapeutic diet is necessarily, make the switch gradually. Mix with the "regular" diet for the first several days to slowly introduce the change, and then increase the percentage of therapeutic diet day by day.

couldn't find her," says Pam. "Zoë was inside the kitchen cabinet, door closed, sitting on top of the bag of food and eating. It was hysterical!"

The dog also knows how to climb the fence in the yard, to look for company—or food. "She goes up one side and over the top, hooks a back leg all the way through the chain link, lowers herself, and then releases her leg," says Pam. "She looks like Mario [video game] going up and coming down. Fence climbing is her forte."

Pam plans to take Zoë for her heartworm treatment within the next few weeks. In the meantime, with the right food and attention, the little dog's personality has blossomed. "She has this little prance; she bounces, kind of like a goat," says Pam. "She's real lively and happy now." Zoë also has learned to like being touched. "She'll pat us with her paw, to say, 'Pet me!' " says Pam.

Glimpses of her past-life personality still surface from time to time. "She's very coy, very canny," says Pam. "You can see the wheels turning. Probably that's why she survived."

Kidney Failure

Kidneys remove toxins and waste from the bloodstream and eliminate them in the urine. They also help regulate fluids in the body and nutrients carried in the blood. "It's kind of like quality control of the body," says Dan Carey, DVM. Kidneys also manufacture various hormones such as erythropoietin, which controls blood pressure and the production of red blood cells.

Failure of the kidneys to do their job causes devastating illness. Kidney failure may come on suddenly due to toxins or injury, but chronic kidney disease creeps up on the dog. It's most common in older dogs, probably as a result of normal wear and tear over a lifetime of use. "Kidney disease is either the number one or number two cause of death in cats and dogs in every study that's been done," says Debbie Davenport, DVM. About 10 percent of all dogs over the age of fifteen develop some degree of kidney disease. "Often, though, their owners are simply unaware of the fact that they have that problem," says Dr. Davenport.

Nephrons are the individual structures of the kidney that are able to independently produce urine. As a normal part of aging, nephrons die and are not replaced. Kidneys are able to function even with significant loss of these nephrons. "Typically when 75 percent or more of the nephrons are lost, that's when we begin to see the real critical problems," says Blake Hawley, DVM.

In renal failure the body is not filtering the blood like it's supposed to. "The kidney allows some things to leak out that should be kept, and keeps some things that should be let go," says Dr. Carey.

SENIOR SYMPTOMS

Typical signs of kidney failure begin gradually, and increase with the progression of the disease.

- Increased urination
- Loss of housetraining
- Increased thirst
- Lethargy
- Loss of appetite
- Weight loss
- Dehydration
- Vomiting
- Diarrhea or constipation
- Mouth sores
- Foul ammonia breath

Various blood and urine tests, in conjunction with the symptoms, will lead to a diagnosis of kidney disease. By checking blood urea nitrogen (BUN) and creatinine levels and comparing them to specific urine gravity, veterinarians can get a good idea about kidney function. "You begin to see an inability for the animal to concentrate its urine," says Dr. Hawley. "And you may see a persistent low urine specific gravity." Further screening of the kidneys by X rays or ultrasound may be necessary.

TREATMENT

Chronic kidney disease cannot be cured, but when caught early, some damage can be reversed and the progression slowed. Medications help normalize the blood, and special therapeutic diets can reduce the workload of the kidneys.

Kidney failure often results in severe dehydration, and fluid therapy not only improves the dog's physical status but also makes a difference in quality of life. "If the animal needs fluids there is no single thing you can do for them that's greater than rehydrating them," says Susan Wynn, DVM.

She also recommends certain natural therapies that seem to improve the animal's quality of life. "There are some herbs that are pretty amazing," she says. "A Chinese herbal formula called Liu Wei Di Huang Wan really does seem to help some of these animals live longer, feel better, and it just seems to be the little extra something that some of them need." The herbal combination also is known by the brand names Six Flavor Tea Pills or Rehmannia Six. These are prescription medications that are available only through your holistic veterinarian.

Dr. Wynn also recommends supplementing the dog's diet with fish oil, which some evidence suggests may slow the degeneration of the kidneys. That's because kidney failure results when each individual nephron develops high blood pressure within the kidney. "That increased blood pressure is considered to be one of the factors that progresses the disease," says Dr. Carey.

ACE inhibitors (angiotensin converting enzymes) such as enalapril and lisinopril, often used to treat heart disease, also help control blood pressure that causes damage to the kidneys. Omega-3 fatty acids (found in fish oil) also reduce the blood pressure within each tiny filter unit. Omega-3 fatty acids are available in health food stores.

Many of the waste products in the blood that make the dog feel bad are from protein metabolism. Again, therapeutic diets are designed to address this concern. "The level of protein [in a therapeutic diet] is typically going to be lower, but of a very high quality and very high digestibility," says Dr. Davenport. "Protein and phosphorus are linked together, so when you try to control dietary phosphorus you also reduce dietary protein."

Another waste product in the blood is nitrogen. Researchers have found that the normal bacteria in the intestine will use nitrogen to replace their cell walls. "If you give the bacteria a food source like a fermentable fiber, it

FEEDING FOR HEALTH

Dogs can suffer different degrees of kidney failure, and may prefer one food over another. Some of the more common therapeutic diets available from your veterinarian for kidney disease include:

- Eukanuba Veterinary Diets, Nutritional Kidney Formula Early Stage
- Eukanuba Veterinary Diets, Nutritional Kidney Formula Advanced Stage
- Hill's Prescription Diet Canine g/d (early stage)
- Hill's Prescription Diet Canine k/d (moderate stage)
- Hill's Prescription Diet Canine u/d (advanced stage)
- IVD Select Canine Modified Formula
- Purina Veterinary Diets, NF Kidney Function Formula
- Waltham Canine Renal Support and Early Renal Support Diets

will grab the nitrogen from the urea, put it into the cell wall, and it can't get back into the bloodstream," says Dr. Carey. "You can shift the excretion from the kidney to the intestine enough to help the body."

Nearly all the major pet food companies offer therapeutic diets for kidney disease, and most have one for "early stage" and another for the more advanced disease. Most restrict phosphorus and sodium, and provide a low to moderate level of highly digestible protein to help relieve the burden on the organs. Some increase omega-3 fatty acids to help reduce hypertension, along with additional B vitamins and others to replace those lost.

Sick dogs often lose their appetite, which can exacerbate the problem. Finding a kidney diet they'll eat is much more important than a particular brand. Don't hesitate to ask for another option if your dog refuses the first diet.

HEMODIALYSIS

Dialysis is standard medical treatment for human patients with chronic renal failure. A machine takes the place of the damaged kidneys, and cleanses the blood of the toxins. Although the technology has been available for many years, it wasn't until 1998 that a program for pets was launched at University of California—Davis. "We use neonatal equipment, and we can accommodate dogs and cats as small as two kilograms," says Larry Cowgill, DVM, an internist at Cal-Davis and founder of the program.

Hemodialysis is used primarily for acute (sudden onset) kidney failure, to give the organs time to heal. "Usually an animal will die of acute kidney failure in four to five days, but it may take weeks or even months for the kidney to [heal]," says Dr. Cowgill. In the past, these dogs were either euthanized or made comfortable during the time it took for them to die. He says, "But now many of those animals have correctable diseases if you can just keep them alive long enough."

Dogs with chronic kidney failure are usually not good candidates for dialysis, because the process is so expensive, and they would need treatment for the rest of their lives. In rare instances in which the dog is a candidate for a kidney transplant, though, hemodialysis can stabilize them before and after surgery until the new organ starts to work.

Hemodialysis units for pets are available in only a handful of places, including the University of California Veterinary Medical Center—San Diego at the Helen Woodward Animal Medical Center in Rancho Santa Fe, the Animal Medical Center in New York, and Tufts University in Boston.

TRANSPLANTS

Jonathan F. McAnulty, DVM, an associate professor of surgery at the University of Wisconsin, began transplanting kidneys in pets in 1995, and like other researchers, finds that there are some real stumbling blocks to dog transplants. "The primary one is that nobody has yet devised a way to consistently prevent rejection in dogs," he says. "The actual placing of the organ and getting it to work is a piece of cake. But managing that case so they don't reject that organ after a period of months is very difficult."

Antirejection drugs such as cyclosporine are used successfully in people (and cats), but they don't work well in dogs, in part because they metabolize the drug differently. Dogs also just seem to be hypersensitive to foreign tissue, probably because of the myriad of blood types in the dog. When surgery is done, it is expensive, and antirejection medication will be needed for the rest of the dog's life. The larger the dog the bigger the dose, and the greater the bill for this medicine, says Dr. McAnulty.

The best matches come from a littermate or offspring of the dog needing the transplant. Kidney transplant technology may offer better options for dogs in the future. Currently, the surgery is considered experimental and is offered in only a handful of universities.

BOTTOM LINE

- "The typical cost for hemodialysis here [University of California—Davis] is about $300 to $400 per treatment," says Dr. Cowgill. During the course of treatment that can easily run to $5,000 to $7,000.
- Kidney transplant costs $6,000 to $8,000 at the University of Wisconsin, and antirejection medicines following surgery typically cost about $1,500 per year for maintenance.

Golden Moments: A Doozer of a Dog

Nancy Lind of Chicago has been active in canine competition for many years. She is also affiliated with Rainbow Animal Assisted Therapy, and says the work has helped keep her mature dogs feeling young and important. "Dogs like a job. They need to do something," says Nancy.

Black-and-tan miniature Dachshund Doozer came to live with Nancy at age two. By the time Doozer was twelve, Nancy had retired her from agility, flyball, and obedience competition. "Her fading eyesight was interfering with her competing," says Nancy.

But Doozer continues her work as a therapy dog, and at fourteen she remains the undisputed queen dog in charge of Nancy's other two dogs. "I'm sure she's still feeling pretty good, because she takes great pleasure in chasing the puppy [a Dachshund mix] out of the room," says Nancy. "She's trying to keep Beaner in his place."

There have been a few changes over the years. "She's no longer black and tan; she's black and white," says Nancy. She won't roll over anymore—probably because of a stiff back. "And now that she's fourteen she loves for me to carry her up and down the stairs—she *allows* me to. She did stairs for thirteen years, though, and refused to be carried."

Doozer works as a therapy dog twice a month in a hospital. Up until this past year, the dog had no problem walking down the long hallways on her way in and out of the sessions. Then Nancy noticed it was getting tougher, so she began to carry Doozer. "I want her to use her energy for the forty-five- to fifty-five-minute sessions with the kids," she says. "She doesn't like being carried in, but she doesn't mind being carried out—those sessions can be tiring!"

Doozer has always been really good with kids, and the therapy groups include any age, from preschoolers to teenagers. The dog follows the directions the child gives and does tricks like jumping through hoops, pushing a car, fetching, giving paw, waving—all the typical activities, says Nancy. Doozer has been at this for so long, she knows she's supposed to follow their

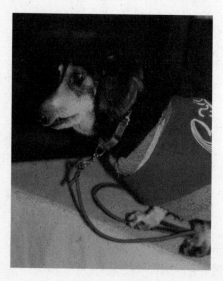

Doozer's kidney disease doesn't stop her from working as a therapy dog. *(Photo Credit: Amy D. Shojai)*

commands—but there is some "trained disobedience" built into the therapy. "If they don't give the command quite right—not moving their arms up far enough or talking loud enough—the dog will look at them and say, 'You're not doing them good enough.' That helps the kids in their therapy," says Nancy.

Doozer will continue doing therapy work for as long as she enjoys it and her health continues to be good. Despite diminished sight, she's not had any trouble getting around the house. Nancy says she's not had her to the ophthalmologist because the dog seems to be functioning fine and her poor sight hasn't seemed to be an inconvenience. She still takes Doozer along to shows when the weather is good. "She's just so happy to be out and doing this, she feels very important then," says Nancy.

Doozer has been diagnosed with early-stage kidney disease. "She's on the early-stage diet," says Nancy, "and takes an antibiotic because she seems to get chronic urinary-tract infections." Other than that, the dog's health remains very good, and her quality of life is outstanding. "To see her run around here, you'd think she was two!" says Nancy.

In fact, Doozer recently wowed the crowd when she outperformed dogs much younger than herself. "I had her at the Doxie Picnic," says Nancy, "and in the Doxie Race she made all those young whippersnappers take a look at her. When I called her, she took off like a shot!" Doozer placed second in a field of young dogs. Although she's a senior-citizen dog, nobody told Doozer she should slow down. She's still having the time of her life.

Liver Disease

The liver acts as an organic processing plant that removes toxins, metabolizes drugs, and manufactures and processes nutrients and enzymes. Liver disease refers to any condition that interferes with one or more of the organ's functions. That can happen to dogs of any age. Because older dogs are more prone to other health challenges, the liver may be more susceptible to stress, damage, or disease in senior canines.

"There is a huge functional reserve to the liver, a lot of backup," says Cynthia R. Leveille-Webster, DVM. Even when a large percentage of the liver stops working, the remainder is able to handle the job. "The other key thing about the liver is that after some insults, it's fully capable of regenerating to its original size," says Dr. Webster. But it takes lots of medical support to buy the necessary time for recovery. And in some disease states, the liver's regenerative capacity becomes limited, and it can't repair itself.

Because the liver interacts with so many other body systems, it can be affected by other conditions, especially Cushing's disease. The excessive production of cortisol associated with Cushing's disease stimulates the liver to make a lot of glycogen—carbohydrate storage material—and so the liver gets really big. Liver tests fall into the abnormal range. "But the liver is actually absolutely fine," says Dr. Webster. "It's just the cortisol inducing all these changes." Once you get Cushing's disease under control, the liver's size returns to normal.

The most common old-dog liver problem is cancer. In particular, a tumor called hemangiosarcoma, which usually originates in the spleen, often spreads to the liver. Drug-induced liver problems are also common, and any drug could cause problems. "Rimadyl [an arthritis medicine] seems to do it more than other drugs," says Dr. Webster, "and older dogs tend to get arthritis, so they're the ones that are on those medications. Long-term use of phenobarbital is another one." Dogs with epilepsy may be given Phenobarbital to control seizures, and after years and years of using the medicine, it may impact the liver. Nonspecific inflammation of the liver—referred to as hepatitis—may also flare up in older dogs.

SENIOR SYMPTOMS

Signs of liver problems are very similar and quite vague, whatever the type of disease.

- Jaundice—yellowish tinge to the gums, whites of eyes, or inside of ears
- Refusal to eat
- Vomiting
- Diarrhea
- Weight loss
- Lethargy
- Swollen abdomen (ascites)
- Ulcers
- Bloody urine or stool
- Neurological signs, including confusion or dullness, known as hepatic encephalopathy

---

DIAGNOSIS

Signs of disease are so vague, more sophisticated tests are required to diagnose liver disease. Bile produced by the liver aids in the digestion of fat, and when it backs up in the blood circulation it can turn the dog's skin yellow. Increased pressure on the veins entering the liver can prompt an accumulation of fluid (ascites), causing the abdomen to swell. Dogs with liver disease often develop ulcers, which can result in bloody urine or feces.

A biochemical profile of the blood is the first step toward diagnosis. Liver enzymes may be elevated for a number of reasons, though, and elevated enzyme values do not automatically mean the dog has liver disease. For instance, dogs with Cushing's disease often have elevated liver enzymes. Blood tests may be followed by ultrasound and possibly a biopsy.

Diagnosis can be complicated by the presence of nodular regeneration, says Dr. Webster. This is a poorly understood mechanism whereby the liver develops little nodules as a result of decreased blood flow. "Sometimes the liver can be peppered with these, and on an ultrasound they look like little cancers," she says. The bumpy liver is simply a sign of aging, and usually doesn't indicate any disease.

Together, blood tests, imaging techniques (ultrasound), and symptoms can point to liver disease. However, a definitive diagnosis can be made only by a biopsy—examining tissue beneath the microscope. An ultrasound-guided needle allows cells to be collected through the abdominal wall, often without invasive surgery.

NURSE ALERT!

Liver disease in older dogs tends to become chronic, and may require long-term care to help the dog maintain a good quality of life.

- Dogs with liver disease are often reluctant to eat. A feeding tube placed surgically in the dog's stomach through the body wall provides the conduit for temporary nutrition. A soft, semiliquid diet given by syringe through the tube maintains nutrition until the dog regains his appetite. Owners may be required to tube-feed the convalescing dog for days to weeks.
- A number of oral medications, usually pills, are often necessary to relieve the symptoms of liver disease.

TREATMENT

Treatment depends on the cause of the problem and how early it's caught. Once the liver scars, the disease is hard to reverse. "The earlier you intervene, the better you can prevent damage," says Dr. Webster.

If the liver problems are caused by drug toxicity, the solution is to stop using the drug. "Many times that is enough to reverse the changes," says Dr. Webster. Hepatitis is usually treated with medicines to try to suppress the inflammation. An oral ursodeoxycholic acid (UDCA, Actigall, or Urso-diol) is a naturally occurring bile acid that helps protect the liver from further damage.

A new supplement on the market, S-Adenosylmethionine (SAMe), is a kind of nutraceutical antioxidant that can increase the antioxidant glutathione levels in liver cells of both dogs and cats. Glutathione is a potent antioxidant that protects liver cells from toxins and death. Recent studies indicate that up to 45 percent of dogs with severe liver problems are deficient in glutathione. Taking S-Adenosylmethionine (brand name Denosyl SD4) has been demonstrated to improve liver function in these pets.

Treatment often involves finding the right balance among medications that address the liver disease, avoid the potential for ulcers, and still manage other existing health concerns such as arthritis. "That's often a big consideration in my elderly patients that have chronic hepatitis," says Dr. Webster, who often suggests replacing arthritis medications in liver-diseased dogs with nutraceuticals such as Cosequin, or recommends acupuncture as an alternative.

When dogs have ulcers, it hurts them to eat. Just the presence of the fluid in the belly also makes them uncomfortable. Medications such as spironolactone act as a diuretic to get rid of the excess belly fluid (ascites) and relieve the discomfort.

Refusing to eat makes sick dogs even sicker and delays recovery. Occasionally force-feeding is necessary to get the dog over the hump. A feeding tube may be placed down the nose into the stomach, or surgically through the dog's side, to allow him to be fed a soft diet, either while in the hospital or after going home.

Once the dog begins eating again on his own, the right diet helps maintain sick dogs and helps them recover. The nutrient profiles of therapeutic diets provide highly digestible protein, zinc, and other ingredients designed to reduce the workload of the liver, support liver repair and regeneration, and help regulate the metabolism of blood sugar.

FEEDING FOR HEALTH

Foods designed to be highly palatable and digestible are appropriate for dogs suffering from liver disease.

- Eukanuba Veterinary Diets, Nutritional Stress/Weight Gain Formula, Maximum-Calorie
- Hill's Prescription Diet Canine a/d (recovery)
- Hill's Prescription Diet Canine l/d (liver diet)
- IVD Selected Care Modified Formula
- Purina Veterinary Diets, EN Gastroenteric Formula
- Waltham Canine Convalescence Support Diets
- Waltham Canine Hepatic Support Diet

Obesity

Any dog can become overweight, but obesity—body fat that's 20 percent beyond the ideal—more often affects middle-aged and older dogs. It is the most common nutritional disorder of dogs. A recent study of more than twenty-three thousand dogs seen at sixty private veterinary hospitals in thirty states indicated that 40 to 50 percent of dogs aged five to twelve years were overweight, says Sharon A. Center, DVM, an internist and professor of medicine at Cornell University.

The increase in weight problems is caused by a combination of factors. First, dogs are rarely as active as in the past, when they worked on farms and led a predominantly outdoor lifestyle. Spaying and neutering is estimated to induce a 15 to 20 percent reduction in metabolic rate due to the influence of lost sex hormones on appetite and overall reduced activity. Unless food intake and exercise are adjusted, dogs easily gain weight. Today, couch-potato dogs are fed high-calorie, tasty foods, and often overeat either out of boredom or from being overtreated by owners.

Changes in the pet's lifestyle can also impact weight gain. Examples include families moving to a smaller home with limited outside access for the dog; arthritis that reduces the dog's desire to exercise; medications for chronic disease that may cause sedation; and respiratory or heart conditions that interfere with the dog's ability to get around.

Some dogs are more prone to obesity than others, suggesting there is a "fat gene" in dogs. Prone breeds include Labrador Retrievers, Cairn Terriers, Cocker Spaniels, Dachshunds, Cavalier King Charles Spaniels, Shetland

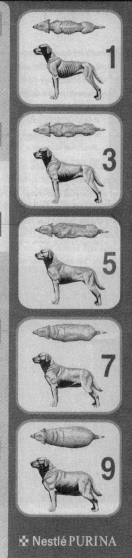
(Reprinted by permission)

Sheepdogs, Basset Hounds, Beagles, Jack Russell Terriers, and Corgis. Dogs that develop hypothyroidism suffer from a slower metabolism that can cause obesity. Also, there is usually a reduction in muscle tissue as dogs age, which reduces the amount of food energy requirements, says Dr. Center.

Dogs don't particularly care how they look, so vanity is not an issue with overweight. Much more important, obesity increases the risk for a number of other health problems, especially for aging dogs. For instance, obesity can quadruple the dog's risk for diabetes, says Dottie LaFlamme, DVM. "It's not going to cause heart problems," she says, "but obesity is an aggravating factor if you have heart problems. Arthritic problems are very much aggravated by excess body weight." Long-term studies also indicate that fat dogs don't live as long as thin ones, so obesity becomes a longevity and quality-of-life issue.

COMFORT ZONE

When put on a diet, dogs often pester owners endlessly asking for more and more food. Try placing a portion of the dog's rations inside one of the commercial puzzle toys. That way, she must work to move the ball to shake out the food. That keeps her from pestering you, keeps her mind engaged, and also encourages her to exercise. A number of puzzle toys are available in pet products outlets.

- Buster Cube, one of the first canine puzzle toys, and still a favorite
- Milk Bone Biscuit Ball is a hard rubber ball with bone-shaped cutouts to wedge treats in. It's made by the Kong Company—there are many varieties of Kong puzzle products for dogs

---

DIAGNOSIS

Weight by itself isn't the best way to evaluate the overweight dog. A much better measure is a hands-on approach in which someone looks at the dog's profile and palpates, or feels, the body composition. Weight gain can happen so gradually that owners may be caught by surprise when the veterinarian suggests the dog is overweight. Other times, people simply aren't familiar with the "ideal" canine physique and don't know that their dog falls outside these parameters.

Some breeds call for slightly different compositions—for instance, Greyhounds and other coursing breeds are supposed to have visible ribs. In general, however, you should be able to feel your dog's ribs, but not see them. From above, you should see a decided break at the waist, beginning at the back of the ribs to just before the hips. The degree of this "hourglass figure" varies somewhat by breed. For example, the Westie will be more level, while the Whippet is quite extreme without being underweight.

In profile, the dog should have a distinct tummy tuck beginning just behind the last ribs and going up into the hind legs. If you can't feel the dog's ribs, and/or she has a pendulous or bulging tummy, your dog is too pudgy. Overweight dogs often develop rolls of fat on the lower back above the tail. To evaluate your dog's condition, compare her appearance to the illustrations in the Body Condition System chart. Remember to account for fur, which can hide pounds.

Before beginning a diet, your veterinarian should examine your dog to rule out hypothyroidism or address other health conditions. Controlling hypothyroidism will often help correct the weight problem as well. The veterinarian will calculate how much weight should be lost, and suggest a diet and exercise plan appropriate to your specific dog. Usually the target is to lose about 1 to 1½ percent of her starting weight per week.

FEEDING FOR HEALTH

Some dogs are able to lose weight simply by reducing the amount of their regular diet and increasing exercise. Most dogs, though, need the extra help of a reduced-calorie food. Some "lite" products are available in grocery stores, but obese dogs usually do best on a therapeutic diet dispensed from the veterinarian. Products designed for canine reducing diets include:

- Eukanuba Veterinary Diets, Nutritional Weight Maintenance Formula, Senior Plus/Canine
- Eukanuba Veterinary Diets, Nutritional Weight Loss Formulas, Restricted-Calorie/Canine
- Hill's Prescription Diet Canine r/d
- Hill's Prescription Diet Canine w/d
- IVD Select Care Canine Hifactor Formula
- IVD Select Care Canine Vegetarian Formula
- Nutro Max Weight Control Formula
- Precise Light Formula for Less Active or Overweight Dogs
- Purina Veterinary Diets, OM Overweight Management Formula
- Waltham Canine Calorie Control Diet

TREATMENT

Exercise is important not only to maintain weight or prevent further weight gain, but also to take off the extra pounds. For good health, dogs need twenty minutes of aerobic exercise twice a day.

Obese dogs will not be able to sustain high-energy activities for a very long time, and it's important to ease into any type of exercise program. Controlled leash walking is ideal. Simply walk at the dog's pace and build up her stamina. As the weight comes off, her energy level will increase. Start with a ten-minute walk in the morning and afternoon, and add another five minutes each week. Once the dog is able to walk for twenty minutes at a stretch, try picking up the pace and increasing the distance. The interaction you share with your dog during the walk is much healthier for you both than giving her attention with a treat.

Very overweight dogs may be reluctant to move at all. "Make the animals work a little bit for their food," suggests Sarah K. Abood, DVM. "Your animal can't handle a flight of stairs, so how about a ramp up to a chair so they're expending a few calories. For pets that are more ambulatory, put the food at the top or bottom of the staircase so the animal always has to go up and down some stairs to get her food."

Moderately overweight dogs may shed pounds simply by cutting out the treats and increasing exercise. Leaving dry food out for all-day munching rarely works for weight-reduction, so measured meals is recommended. Senior diets typically have fewer calories, and switching the dog to a more age-specific formula can be quite helpful.

AGE-DEFYING TIPS

Keeping the dog slim from an early age will prevent health problems, help her live longer, and increase her enjoyment of life.

- Make twice-daily exercise part of your routine.
- Reward with attention, not treats.
- Choose an age- and activity-appropriate diet. Pets that sleep on the sofa all day do not need the equivalent of rocket fuel. Feeding guidelines listed on pet food packages are a *starting point only*, and tend to be too generous—adjust the amount fed to your dog based on his individual needs.
- Feed measured amounts in meals instead of free-feeding from an ever-full bowl of food.

Another option is to switch the dog to a "lite" formula diet. Just be aware that the lite designation only means the food is lower in calories than the same-brand "regular" food—it's a comparison within the same family of foods. Switching pet food companies may mean a lite food has more calories than the dog's regular diet.

Divide the food into four or even five small meals a day to help keep your dog from feeling deprived. Multiple small meals also tend to increase the body's metabolic rate, so she burns more calories faster and consequently loses the excess weight.

When the dog is obese, medical supervision by the veterinarian and often a special therapeutic weight-loss diet is necessary. Several are available from different pet food manufacturers, and each offers innovative formulations that help the dog safely lose weight. For instance, added vitamins and amino acids such as L-carnitine help get fat molecules into the cells to be burned, says Dan Carey, DVM. "We've also noticed that when overweight animals are reduced in weight with a diet containing L-carnitine, they maintain a whole lot more muscle mass than they do if they have the exact same diet without L-carnitine," he says.

Senility

All dogs tend to suffer some memory loss as they age. A percentage of old dogs develop more severe symptoms, technically called Canine Cognitive Dysfunction, which could be compared to human senility. The older the dog is the more likely he is to show impairment in this area.

"These dogs remind people of a relative or friend with Alzheimer's," says Benjamin Hart, DVM, a veterinary behaviorist at the University of California-Davis. Studies by Dr. Hart and others at the University of California-Davis published in 2001 showed that 30 percent of dogs aged 11 to 12 had one or more symptom, and 68 percent of the 15 to 16 year old dogs had one or more symptom—35 percent of this group had two or more symptoms. Castrated male dogs were significantly more likely to have problems with disorientation than spayed females, but there were no differences between the sexes in other categories.

"Nine years old is sort of when they really start to develop brain pathology," says William Milgram, PhD. "Then the older they are, the more pathology you see, the more severe their cognitive dysfunction." He says that dogs are one of the few species that develop a beta amyloid pathology in the brain. Beta amyloid is a starchlike protein that becomes waxy once deposited in the brain tissues. "Beta amyloid occurs in the human brain as well," says Dr. Milgram. It has been associated with Alzheimer's disease in people.

SENIOR SYMPTOMS

Signs of Canine Cognitive Dysfunction can be vague and confusing, and mimic other disease conditions. Look for:

- Disorientation: wanders aimlessly, acts lost and confused, may not recognize family members or other familiar people or places, gets "stuck" in corners or lost in the house
- Interaction changes: no longer greets family members, dislikes or avoids petting, not as interested in getting attention, interaction changes with other pets
- Sleep changes: is awake and active at night, sleep cycles are disrupted or reversed
- Housetraining is forgotten
- Anxiety or compulsive behaviors: tremors, howling, repetitive pacing, licking the floor or other objects, circling, tail chasing

---

In his studies, Dr. Milgram is imaging the brains of live dogs using an MRI to evaluate changes in the aging canine. "With human Alzheimer's you get these huge ventricles—spaces inside the brain that contain fluid. These spaces become really enlarged in the brains of people with certain types of neurological disorders because there's a lot of cell death," he says. Basically, the brain shrinks and these ventricles become bigger. "We also see that in these really old dogs."

COMFORT ZONE

Dogs suffering from senility often forget to ask to go outside, and have accidents in the house. Keeping the dog's bedding and your carpet and upholstery clean and odor-free helps maintain quality of life for you both.

- Nature's Fresh spray (made by Nature's Sunshine) contains natural proteins derived from vegetable sources and fruit acids to neutralize organic odors due to urine, feces, and vomit, and helps prevent or remove stains. It is safe to spray into the air or on any material not harmed by water (shoes, clothing, bed linens, upholstery, carpet, auto interiors, etc). Nature's Fresh with sprayer costs about $9 and is available at www.vir-chew-all.com
- Tuff Oxi (Tuff Products for Pets) is an enzymatic cleaner that "digests" the smell and organic particles to eliminate odor, and is available from info@tuffcleaningproducts.com

Getting lost in the house or yard, going to the wrong door, forgetting how to signal to go outdoors for urination or defecation—these and other signs correlate with some of the age-related degenerative changes in the dog's brain that are involved with memory and learning, says Dr. Hart. "The deposition of beta amyloid material is somewhat different in the dogs than in the humans. In the dogs it's very diffuse and doesn't consolidate into distinct plaques as it does in humans. But when you see this in humans, the most marked pathological sign is Alzheimer's."

AGE-DEFYING TIPS

In studies of the new Hill's b/d food, researchers found that mental stimulation drastically improved the cognitive function of aging dogs. "It wasn't just food," says Dr. Lansberg. "It was food plus the mental stimulation that greatly enhanced their cognitive function compared to the animals that didn't have the food and those that didn't have the activity."

- Keep your dog both physically active and mentally engaged throughout his life to keep his brain young and to prevent or slow the progression of aging changes. Teach him obedience or trick training.
- Offer puzzle toys that reward his interaction by dispensing treats. The "Talk to Me Treatball" (available at PETsMART) is a hard plastic ball that both holds treats and has a tape recorder for the owner's taped messages to help keep the dog engaged.
- The best rewards are treats or toys the dog adores that are offered only during training. Many dogs (and owners) give high marks to Liver Biscotti, an all-natural crunchy treat available at www.liverbiscotti.com.

TREATMENT

It's important to diagnose cognitive dysfunction correctly. Behavior changes in the aging dog often have other causes. For example, a break in housetraining might be due to kidney disease or diabetes, while disorientation and personality changes could be caused by a brain tumor, or neurological disruptions from liver disease.

When the symptoms are caused by cognitive disorder, owners typically put their elderly dogs to sleep. Surveys of veterinarians indicate that in the United States, up to 500,000 dogs with cognitive disorder are put to sleep each year. However, there is now medical help that can reverse the

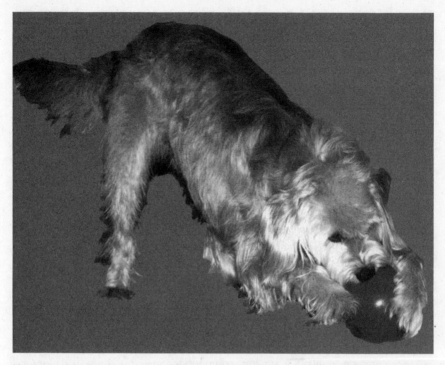

Keep your dog's mind active with games and puzzle toys. They help exercise him and prevent obesity and also can slow down the brain aging that causes Alzheimer's-like symptoms. *(Photo Credit: 2002 Talk to Me™ Pet Products)*

condition in a percentage of affected dogs, and preserve the bond between the owners and their pets.

The human medicine selegiline hydrochloride (Anipryl) has been FDA-approved to treat Canine Cognitive Disorder. Anipryl may work to prevent ongoing damage to the brain. "It acts on one of the neurotransmitters in the brain responsible for nerve-to-nerve communication," says Bill Fortney, DVM. "The drug slows the natural destruction of the chemical compound dopamine in the brain."

The medicine won't work in all cases, however. "In about one third of dogs who have this syndrome, Anipryl works spectacularly, amazingly, and people can't believe it," says Nicholas Dodman, BVMS. "In one-third it produces improvements that are worthwhile. And in one-third it doesn't do anything at all."

Because the problem is progressive, even if the drug works at first, ulti-mately it will stop being effective. "The medicine is not a magical elixir or fountain of youth," says Dr. Dodman. "It does reverse aging changes in a percentage of dogs, for a period of time, but the end is inevitable."

Even in dogs that benefit from the drug, there will be an eventual decline of cognitive function. "It can buy a lot of dogs a lot of time," says Dr. Dodman. "A year or two is a lot of time in a dog's life." Dogs will need to be on the drug for about four weeks before any results can be expected.

Dr. Hart conducted a study comparing cognitive function of neutered to intact male dogs. His results suggest that testosterone present in the aging sexually intact dogs slowed the progression of cognitive impairment, especially among those dogs who were already showing mild symptoms. He expects to get similar results when he compares spayed to intact female dogs. Therefore, he says hormone replacement therapy—testosterone for neutered males and estrogen for spayed females—could prove to be a helpful treatment to delay the onset of memory loss in aging dogs.

COMFORT ZONE

A natural component of some foods, called phospholipids, can help reverse some signs of cognitive disorders by helping brain cells send and receive nerve impulses more effectively. Choline and phosphatidylcholine, two common message-sending compounds, are found in a dietary supplement called Cholodin, which is a less expensive alternative to Anipryl. The products are available through veterinarians, and come in a pill form or powder to be mixed into the food. More information is available at www.mvplabs.com.

NEW FRONTIERS

A number of other studies have investigated selegiline for its antioxidant properties and influence on longevity. David S. Bruyette, DVM, has researched the survival time of dogs on the therapy, and discovered that longevity was significantly greater in treated dogs compared to those on a placebo. Dogs in the study were ten to fifteen years old, and at the end of the two and-a-quarter year study, 80 percent of the selegiline-treated dogs were alive, compared to only 39 percent of the dogs that received the sugar pill. Interestingly, the most common cause of death in the placebo group was cancer, whereas no dogs in the selegiline group died from tumors. It remains to be seen what impact such studies may have for our aging dogs.

BOTTOM LINE

Depending on the size of the dog, Anipryl costs about $1.50 to $2.50 a day.

The newest treatment was made available in early 2002. Hill's Prescription Diet Canine b/d incorporates a combination of antioxidants to help fight the signs of brain aging in dogs. Eating the diet helps keep the dog's memory sharp, which helps reduce house soiling, improves interaction with the family, and reduces disorientation. The innovative diet is available by prescription from veterinarians.

Stroke

A cerebral vascular accident, called a "stroke" in humans, is a disorder of the blood vessels in the cerebrum (front part of the brain), as a result of an impaired blood supply. "Cerebral vascular accident is something we definitely see in pets," says Lisa Klopp, DVM.

Common causes of stroke in people include smoking, primary high blood pressure, and atherosclerosis, which are deposits of cholesterol-rich plaques within the arteries. Strokes are not as common in animals because pets don't have those diseases, says Dr. Klopp.

In most cases, a cerebral vascular accident in dogs is associated with hypertension (high blood pressure) as a result of kidney failure, infectious disease, or inflammation of the heart (endocarditis). Endocrine diseases like Cushing's disease and hypothyroidism seem to allow predispositions for vascular accident, says Dr. Klopp, but many times an underlying cause can't be found.

DIAGNOSIS

Diagnosis can be difficult. Even with an MRI, the changes caused by the brain damage may be hard to see. "If the stroke is big enough to see in the brain stem, the animal is probably not alive," says Dr. Klopp. "The brain stem is very sensitive and there's no functional redundancy there, so a very small stroke is going to do a lot of damage."

SENIOR SYMPTOMS

Symptoms of a stroke are vague, will be variable, and depend on what part of the brain is affected. "People say, if the animal comes in dizzy it's got to be a stroke—well, no," says Dr. Klopp. "Anything that affects the vestibular area [inner ear] is going to cause dizziness." Symptoms of a stroke are usually very sudden and may be severe, but then usually tend to improve.

- Seizure is by far the most common symptom
- Behavior change (anything!) may also be a sign

However, strokes in the forebrain are easier to see on the MRI. "We can have fairly good-size strokes in the forebrain and have animals survive," says Dr. Klopp. "If I think a stroke is possible, but I'm not seeing signs on the MRI, I try to rule other things out and go from there."

TREATMENT

Once the stroke has occurred, there's not much you can do about it. "By the time I see it, it's probably as bad as it's ever going to be," says Dr. Klopp. "It's happened, the animal's bad, and then typically the animal improves."

Treatment is aimed at supporting the dog and giving him time to recover. If there's an underlying cause, the disease is also treated. If the dog has hypertension, you want to get that under control. When heart disease, endocrine disorders, or other conditions are at the root, the veterinarian may consult with a specialist.

NURSE ALERT!

The aftermath of a stroke may leave your dog very weak, confused, or unable to walk. Recovery time varies, depending on the severity of the damage. But in almost all cases, dogs slowly improve. In the meantime, you may need to offer extra TLC.

- Soften food or hand-feed
- Carry him to the outdoor "facilities," or provide absorbent pads in his bed to help deal with accidents
- Rehabilitation exercises may help strengthen weak muscles
- Medicate as indicated to deal with underlying diseases

Dogs tend to recover more easily from strokes than people do. "I've seen very badly affected animals walk out of the hospital," says Dr. Klopp. "Part of it is they don't feel sorry for themselves; they don't have to drive a car; they don't have to sit down and play piano; they just have to be a pet," she says. Dogs are very good at compensating. If they have a weakness in one or more legs, they adjust and walk more slowly or carefully on stairs, for example.

Also, dogs are much more dependent on their brain stem for their strength and function than people. If they have a stroke in the forebrain they may initially be very weak, but they'll usually get up and get going again with only a few subtle deficits. "They're not going to be paralyzed on one side like the human," says Dr. Klopp.

Urinary Incontinence

There are many reasons why a dog might have a lapse in housetraining. Behavioral issues often have to do with territorial marking, or with inadequate training where the dog simply doesn't know any better. These tend not to be age-related.

An increased urge to urinate develops with diseases such as diabetes and kidney failure, which are more common in senior dogs. In these cases, treating the underlying problem reduces the symptom. Finally, cognitive dysfunction may prompt increased accidents when the old dog's brain simply forgets the training, or can't find the way to the proper spot.

Urinary incontinence, though, refers specifically to a loss of bladder control. "Some of these things are just aging changes, and they may not be able to control their bladders as well as they used to," says Rhonda Schulman, DVM.

SENIOR SYMPTOMS

Urinary incontinence due to age typically happens unconsciously and is a physical problem.

- Wetting when relaxed or resting
- Wetting while asleep
- Urine scald (similar to diaper rash) around genitals

"Old spayed dogs have a problem like postmenopausal women," says Tracy Ridgeway, DVM, a general-practice veterinarian in Washington. In most cases, these dogs are incontinent only when they're sleeping, and they are unaware of the leakage. "It seems to be due to a lack of estrogen," says Dr. Schulman. "Their bladder sphincter gets fairly incompetent." The decline in the hormone causes a decrease in the muscle tone that controls the urethra. More rarely, castrated males have a similar problem. Large and giant-breed dogs, obese dogs, and dogs with docked tails (especially Old English Sheepdogs, Rottweilers, Dobermans, and Weimaraners) are affected most often.

NURSING ALERT!

If your dog develops urinary incontinence, it's more than an inconvenience. It can also be a health problem that requires ongoing nursing care.

- Watch for urine scald—red, irritated, burned-looking skin around the genitals—vulva on female dogs and the prepuce that covers the male's penis.
- Keep the area clean with baby wipes or other mild cleansers.
- Protect the skin with Desitin or a triple antibiotic ointment to help prevent infection.

TREATMENT

Accidents most often happen when the dog drinks too much before bedtime and can't "hold it" until the morning bathroom break. "The fuller the bladder, the more the leakage," says Anna Worth, VMD. Just pick up the water bowl two hours before bedtime, and make sure the dog uses the bathroom before you turn in for the night.

In most cases, your veterinarian must prescribe medicine to help control the incontinence by improving the strength of the bladder sphincter. Hormone replacement therapy—testosterone for male dogs, and more commonly estrogen, (diethylstilbestrol, brand names DES and Premarin)—helps some female dogs. It must be given in tiny doses calculated by the veterinarian for your individual dog's needs, says Dr. Ridgeway. The medication is needed for the rest of the dog's life.

Dr. Schulman says the most effective and commonly prescribed drug to improve bladder sphincter control and treat incontinence is phenyl-propanolamine (PPA). PPA was taken off the market when people developed problems from taking it as an ingredient in common diet medications, but dogs don't have those problems, and they still benefit from PPA.

"It's still out there, but harder to find," says Dr. Schulman. "They've now made a veterinary version of it that's chewable, or we just get it compounded." Compounded medication is made by specialized pharmacies on a case-by-case basis for the individual patient, rather than being mass-produced by a pharmaceutical company as a one-size-fits-all product.

Compounding medication not only makes discontinued drugs available, but can also adjust the dose into the tiny amounts necessary for drugs like

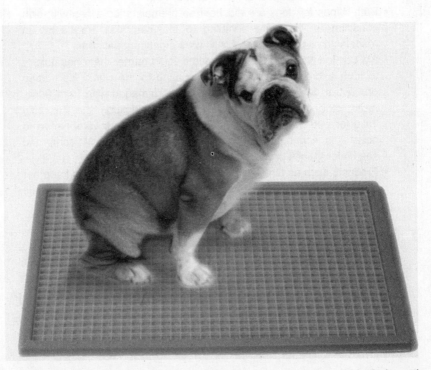

Aging dogs aren't able to maintain control for as long as they could in their youth. When you aren't able to increase the number of bathroom breaks, an alternative is to provide indoor toilet facilities. WizDog provides a grid to keep the pet away from the waste and a tray to catch it, and the grid comes in sizes to accommodate tiny to very large dogs. *(Photo Credit: WizDog Housetraining Toilet)*

DES. Also, compounded medicines can create daily medications in a form that dogs more readily accept, such as an injection, a liver-flavored oral liquid, or even a patch that allows the drug to be absorbed through the skin.

COMFORT ZONE

Save yourself frustration and aggravation by confining the incontinent dog to an easy-to-clean area with linoleum. Or you can protect carpet and furniture by putting down sheets of plastic and spreading disposable diapers or products like Depend undergarments to catch the urine.

- Some pet product stores carry diaperlike products made for dogs, such as Pet Bloomers. They come sized for toy dogs at two to five pounds, and up to extra-large size for 95- to 120-pound dogs, and are available through Drs. Foster and Smith.
- Bath Wipes for dogs are alcohol-free premoistened wipes with skin conditioners. They are soothing to inflamed skin, and come in resealable packages, available at www.eightinonepet.com.
- 3M Cavilon No Sting Barrier Film is a liquid barrier that dries quickly to form a breathable, transparent coating to the skin. This human product is designed to protect intact or damaged skin from urine, feces, other body fluids, tape trauma, and friction—and it is also ideal for pets with incontinence problems. Ask your veterinarian to order this spray product for you, or contact www.3M.com, and search for "health products + incontinence."
- Products such as Dri-Dek elevate the dog from the floor to keep her away from "accidents." The waffle-shaped material comes in sheets that can be fitted to your size needs. Contact www.dri-dek.com.

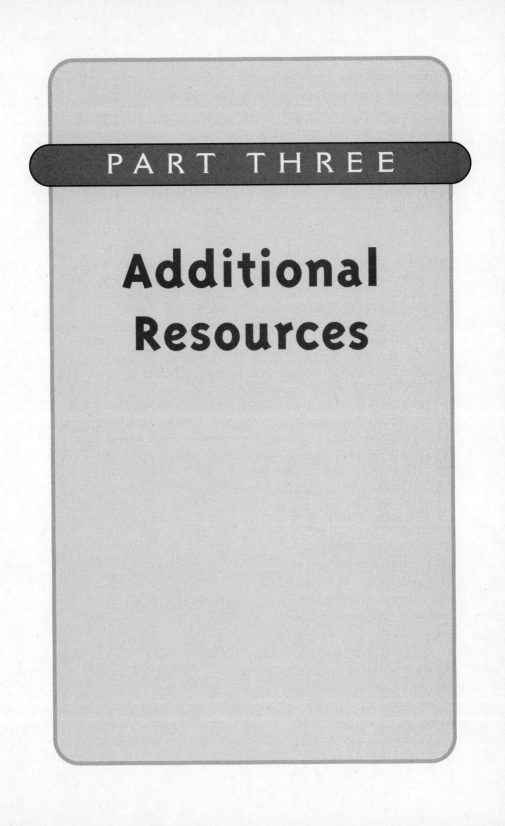

PART THREE

Additional
Resources

Senior-Care Directory

One of the best ways to find out about care options and receive emotional support is to talk with other dog owners who have experienced similar situations with their pets. A good place to start is at the veterinary schools, which often have resources for pet owners on various senior dog conditions, as well as grief counseling services. If you have access to the Internet, go to the various Web sites and do a search on the topic of your choice.

VETERINARY SCHOOLS AND BEREAVEMENT HOT LINES

Alabama

Auburn University
College of Veterinary Medicine
Auburn University, Alabama 36849
www.vetmed.auburn.edu

Tuskegee University
School of Veterinary Medicine
Tuskegee University College of Veterinary Medicine, Nursing, and Allied Health
Tuskegee, Alabama 36088
http://vetmed.tusk.edu

California

University of California
School of Veterinary Medicine
One Shields Avenue
Davis, California 95616
www.vetmed.ucdavis.edu
Grief Hot Line: 800-565-1526

Colorado

Colorado State University
College of Veterinary Medicine
and Biomedical Sciences
Fort Collins, Colorado 80523-1601
www.cvmbs.colostate.edu
Grief Hot Line: 970-491-1242

Florida

University of Florida
College of Veterinary Medicine
P.O. Box 100125
Gainesville, Florida 32610-0125
www.vetmed.ufl.edu
Grief Hot Line: 352-392-4700 ext. 4080

Georgia

University of Georgia
College of Veterinary Medicine
Athens, Georgia 30602
www.vet.uga.edu

Illinois

University of Illinois
College of Veterinary Medicine
2001 South Lincoln
Urbana, Illinois 61802
www.cvm.uiuc.edu
Grief Hot Line: 217-244-2273 or 877-394-2273

Indiana

Purdue University
School of Veterinary Medicine
1240 Lynn Hall
West Lafayette, Indiana 47907-1240
www.vet.purdue.edu

Iowa

Iowa State University
College of Veterinary Medicine
Christensen Drive
Ames, Iowa 50011-1250
www.vetmed.iastate.edu
Grief Hot Line: 888-478-7574

Kansas

Kansas State University
College of Veterinary Medicine
101 Trotter Hall
Manhattan, Kansas 66506-5601
www.vet.ksu.edu

Louisiana

Louisiana State University
School of Veterinary Medicine
Skip Bertman Drive
Baton Rouge, Louisiana 70803
www.vetmed.lsu.edu
Grief Hot Line: 225-578-9547

Massachusetts

Tufts University
School of Veterinary Medicine
200 Westboro Road
North Grafton, Massachusetts 01536
www.tufts.edu/vet
Grief Hot Line: 508-839-7966

Michigan

Michigan State University
College of Veterinary Medicine
G100 Vet Med Center
East Lansing, Michigan 48824-1316
www.cvm.msu.edu
Grief Hot Line: 517-432-2696

Minnesota

The University
of Minnesota
College of Veterinary Medicine
410 Veterinary Teaching Hospital
St. Paul, Minnesota 55108
www.cvm.umn.edu

Mississippi

Mississippi State University
College of Veterinary Medicine
Box 9825
Mississippi State, Mississippi 39762-9825
www.cvm.msstate.edu

Missouri

University of Missouri
College of Veterinary Medicine
Columbia, Missouri 65211
www.cvm.missouri.edu

New York

Cornell University
College of Veterinary Medicine
Box 39, Schurman Hall S3-005
Ithaca, New York 14853-6401
www.vet.cornell.edu
Grief Hot Line: 607-253-3932

North Carolina

North Carolina State University
College of Veterinary Medicine
4700 Hillsborough Street
Raleigh, North Carolina 27606
www.cvm.ncsu.edu/

Ohio

Ohio State University
College of Veterinary Medicine
1900 Coffey Road
Columbus, Ohio 43210
www.vet.ohio-state.edu
Grief Hot Line: 614-292-1823

Oklahoma

Oklahoma State University
College of Veterinary Medicine
110 McElroy Hall
Stillwater, Oklahoma 74078
www.cvm.okstate.edu

Oregon

Oregon State University
College of Veterinary Medicine
200 Magruder Hall
Corvallis, Oregon 97331-4801
www.vet.orst.edu

Pennsylvania

University of Pennsylvania
School of Veterinary Medicine
3800 Spruce Street
Philadelphia, Pennsylvania 19104
www.vet.upenn.edu
Grief Hot Line: 215-898-4529

Tennessee

University of Tennessee
College of Veterinary Medicine
P.O. Box 1071
Knoxville, Tennessee 37996
www.vet.utk.edu

Texas

Texas A&M University
College of Veterinary Medicine
Suite 101-VMA
College Station, Texas 77843-4461
www.cvm.tamu.edu

Virginia

Virginia Tech and University of Maryland
Virginia-Maryland Regional
College of Veterinary Medicine
Duck Pond Drive
Blacksburg, Virginia 24061-0442
www.vetmed.vt.edu
Grief Hot Line: 540-231-8038

Washington

Washington State University
College of Veterinary Medicine
Pullman, Washington 99164-7010
www.vetmed.wsu.edu
Grief Hot Line: 509-335-5704

Wisconsin

University of Wisconsin-Madison
School of Veterinary Medicine
2015 Linden Drive
Madison, Wisconsin 53706-1102
www.vetmed.wisc.edu

WEB SITES AND E-MAIL LISTS

The Internet provides enormous resources in terms of informational Web sites, message boards, live "chats," and E-mail discussion groups. A Web search on any subject, such as "pet loss" or "canine Cushing's" will return a list of helpful resources. It's best to visit the site or read a description before subscribing to an E-mail list or joining in open discussions, to determine if the resource fits your needs. Here are a few to get you started.

General Resources

(Good jumping-off points, search for "dog health" or specific subjects)

www.smartgroups.com
www.topica.com
http://dir.groups.yahoo.com
www.k9web.com/dog-faqs/lists/email-list.html

Addison's Disease

http://groups.yahoo.com/group/k9addisons
http://groups.yahoo.com/group/SA_Addisons

Back Problems

AbleDogs
Primarily for people whose pets (mostly dogs) are experiencing back problems, recovering from surgery (mostly spinal), are paralyzed, in carts, and so forth.
http://groups.yahoo.com/group/abledogs/
www.abledogs.net

Blindness

BLINDDOGS list:
http://groups.yahoo.com/group/blinddogs/

BLIND-DEAF-DOGS list:
http://groups.yahoo.com/group/blind-deaf-dogs

Cancer

http://groups.yahoo.com/group/caninecancer
http://groups.yahoo.com/group/canineswithcancer

Cushing's Disease

www.io.com/~lolawson/cushings/
http://groups.yahoo.com/group/caninecushings-autoimmunecare

CUSHINGS-PETS list.
Subscribe with E-mail to:
listserv@listserv.tamu.edu
with a message in the form: subscribe CUSHINGS-PETS your name
(your pet's name/breed/date of diagnosis)

Deafness

DEAFDOGS list
http://groups.yahoo.com/group/deafdogs/

BLIND-DEAF-DOGS list
http://groups.yahoo.com/group/blind-deaf-dogs

Diabetes Mellitus

PETDIABETES list
Subscribe by E-mailing: majordomo@netwrx1.com
with the message: subscribe PETDIABETES

The Muffin Group (pet diabetes list)
Subscribe with E-mail to: majordomo@netwrx1.com
with the message: subscribe muffin

Epilepsy

EPIL-K9 (epilepsy in dogs)
Subscribe by E-mailing: listserv@apple.ease.lsoft.com
with a message in the form: subscribe EPIL-K9 Yourfirstname Yourlastname

General/Geriatric Pets

VETMED
A moderated discussion list for veterinary medicine and animal health
issues. Veterinary professionals and pet owners are equally welcome to
join.
Subscribe by E-mailing: LISTSERV@IUPUI.EDU
with the message: SUB VETMED Yourfirstname Yourlastname

SENIOR-L (old dogs)
Subscribe by E-mailing: listserv@listserv.aol.com
with the message: subscribe Senior-L Yourname
The Senior Dog Project
www.srdogs.com/Pages/care.fr.html

Kidney Disease

K9KIDNEYS
http://groups.yahoo.com/group/K9KIDNEYS

Pet Loss

Pet Loss Grief Support Web site
www.petloss.com

Association for Pet Loss and Bereavement
www.aplb.org

Finding a Pet Cemetery
International Pet Cemetery Association (referrals)
www.iaopc.com/home.htm

FURTHER READING

Health Care Management

Dog Massage by Maryjean Ballner
St. Martin's Griffin, 2001

Living with a Deaf Dog by Susan Cope Becker
Susan Cope Becker, 1997

Living with Blind Dogs by Caroline D. Levin, RN
Lantern Publications, 1998

The Arthritis Solution for Dogs by Shawn Messonnier, DVM
Prima Publishing, 2000

Natural Health Bible for Dogs and Cats by Shawn Messonnier, DVM
Prima Publishing, 2001

The First-Aid Companion for Dogs and Cats by Amy D. Shojai
Rodale Press, 2001

New Choices in Natural Healing for Dogs and Cats by Amy D. Shojai
Rodale Press, 1999

The Purina Encyclopedia of Dog Care by Amy D. Shojai
Ballantine Books, 1999

Pain Management for the Small Animal Practitioner, by William J. Tranquilli, Kurt A. Grimm, and Leigh A. Lamont
Teton NewMedia, 2000

Bereavement

Coping with Sorrow on the Loss of Your Pet by Moira Allen
Alpine Publishing, 1996

The Loss of a Pet by Wallace Sife
Hungry Minds, Inc., 1998

For Children

A Dog Like Jack by Dyanne Disalvo-Ryan
Holiday House, 1999

Dog Heaven by Cynthia Rylant
Scholastic Trade, 1995

For Every Dog an Angel by Christine Davis
Lighthearted Press, 1997

Mr. Rogers' First Experience: When a Pet Dies by F. Rogers
Paper Star, 1998

INSURANCE AND CARE PLANS

Banfield, The Pet Hospital
"Banfield's Optimum Wellness Plans"
11815 NE Glenn Widing Drive
Portland, OR 97220
Phone: 800-838-6738
Web site: www.vetsmart.com

CareCredit
901 East Cerritos Avenue
Anaheim, CA 92805-6475
Phone: 888-255-4426
Web site: www.carecredit.com

PetAssure
10 South Morris Street
Dover, NJ 07801
Phone: 888-789-7387
Web site: www.petassure.com

PetCare Insurance Programs
P.O. Box 8575
Rolling Meadows, IL 60008-8575
Phone: 866-275-7387
Web site: www.petcareinsurance.com

PetPlan Insurance
777 Portage Avenue
Winnipeg, MB R3G 0N3 Canada
Phone: 1-800-268-1169
Web site: www.petplan.com

Veterinary Pet Insurance
3060 Saturn Street
Brea, CA 92821
Phone: 800-872-7387
Web site: www.petinsurance.com

Vetinsurance
201-557 Southdale Road East
London, ON N6E 1A2
Canada
Phone: 877-838-7387
Web site: www.vetinsurance.com

FOOD FOR SENIORS

Hill's Pet Nutrition
Science Diets and Prescription Diets
www.hillspet.com

Iams Company
Eukanuba, Iams, and Eukanuba Veterinary Diets
www.iams.com

Innovative Veterinary Diets (IVD)
Limited Ingredient Diets, Select Care
www.ivdvetdiets.com

Nestlé Purina PetCare Company
Dog Chow, Purina Veterinary Diets
www.purina.com

Nutro
Natural Choice Dog, Max Dog
www.nutroproducts.com

Precise
www.precisepet.com

Steve's Real Food
(Commercial frozen or freeze-dried raw diet)
www.stevesrealfood.com

Waltham
www.waltham.com

Wysong
www.wysong.net

PRODUCT SOURCES FOR SENIORS

BedderBacks
Dog Bed Ramps
Phone: 877-327-5438
Web site: www.bedderbacks.com

Dewey's Wheelchairs for Dogs
Phone: 877-312-2122
Fax: 877-312-2123
Web site: www.wheelchairsfordogs.com

Drs. Foster and Smith
2253 Air Park Road, P.O. Box 100
Rhinelander, WI 54501
Phone: 800-381-7179
Web site:www.drsfostersmith.com

The Dog's Outfitter
1 Maplewood Drive
Hazleton, PA 18202-9798
Phone: 800-367-3647
Web site: www.dogsoutfitter.com

Dri-Dek Corporation
(Raised grid/floor or kennel liner to keep ill or incontinent dogs clean)
2706 South Horseshoe Drive
Naples, FL 34104
Phone: 800-348-2398
Fax: 800-828-4248
E-mail: info@dri-dek.com
Web site: www.dri-dek.com

Drinkwell Pet Fountain
Veterinary Ventures
5635 Riggins Court, Suite 20
Reno, NV 89502
Phone: 800-805-7532
Web site: www.vetventures.com

K-9 Cart Company
656 SE Bayshore Drive, Suite 2
Oak Harbor, WA 98277
Phone: 360-675-1808, 800-578-6960
Web site: www.k9carts.com

Kong Company
16191-D Table Mountain Parkway
Golden, CO 80403-1641
Phone: 303-216-2626
Web site: www.kongcompany.com

Liver Biscotti
4562 East Second Street, Suite F
Benecia, CA 94510-1410
Phone: 888-500-DOGS (3647) or 707-751-1550
Fax: 707-751-1768
E-mail: info@liverbiscotti.com
Web site: www.liverbiscotti.com

MyEtribute, Inc. provides information and services addressing the
health care and end-of-life needs of senior animals. Features ramps, orthopedic beds, and incontinence pads, specialized greeting cards, gifts,
and burial items.
73415 Pinyon Street
Palm Desert, CA 92260-4711
www.mypettribute.com

Perfect Coat Bath Wipes
Eight in One Pet Products
2100 Pacific Street
Hauppauge, NY 11788
Phone: 800-645-5154
Web site: www.eightinonepet.com

Practivet
Greta Implantable Fluid Tube (GIF-Tube)
2386 GrantsFerry Drive
Biloxi, MS 39531
Phone: 800-535-4057
E-mail: Kristy@practivet.com
Web site: www.practivet.com

Puppy Go Potty
Absorption Corp
1051 Hilton Ave
Bellingham, WA 98225
Phone: 888-Go-Potty (467-6889)
E-mail: dogs@absorption-corp.com
Web site: www.puppygopotty.com

Spillnet Protective Barrier
(protection for floors from pet accidents)
Phone: 800-438-7668
Web site: www.stainmaster.com

Talk to Me Treatball
Phone: 877-860-6227
Web site: www.talktometreatball.com

Tuff Products for Pets
(Tuff Oxi)
4035 Wade Street, Suite B
Los Angeles, CA 90066
Phone: 310-574-3252
E-mail: info@tuffcleaningproducts.com

Vir-Chew-All Enterprizez
(Nature's Fresh Spray)
Phone: 877-695-3750
E-mail: presh@vir-chew-all.com
Web site: www.vir-chew-all.com

WizDog Housetraining Toilet
PETTEK
425 East 51st Street, Suite 8G
New York, NY 10022
E-mail: wizard@wizdog.com
Web site: http://wizdog.com

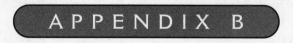

APPENDIX B

HOME MEDICINE CHEST

Human medications are often helpful for dogs, and you may already have many of the following medications in your medicine chest. However, the dosages vary depending on the size of the pet and other ongoing health issues. It's a good idea to keep these products and/or herbs on hand, but it's best to call the veterinarian for a specific dose and medication recommendation for your individual animal.

Medication	*Purpose*
A and D Ointment	Antibacterial ointment for scrapes or wounds
Aloe (herb)	Constipation, skin irritation
Artificial Tears	Eye lubricant
Benadryl	Antihistamine, itch relief, sedative properties
Betadine Solution	Antiseptic soak for cleansing injuries
Bufferin	Pain relief
Burow's Solution	Topical antiseptic
Calendula (herb)	Topical for skin injuries
Chamomile (herb)	Topical skin irritation, tea for stomach problems, stress
Comfrey (herb)	Skin injuries
Dandelion (herb)	Diuretic, for water retention
Desitin	Soothing skin cream
Dulcolax	Constipation

Echinacea (herb)	For infections and inflammation
Eucalyptus (herb)	Nasal congestion
Ginger (herb)	For nausea
Ginkgo (herb)	For mental dullness
Goldenseal (herb)	Infections, bronchial inflammation
Hawthorn (herb)	Heart irregularities
Kaopectate	For diarrhea
Lanacane	Topical anesthetic
Metamucil (unflavored)	For constipation
Milk thistle (herb)	Liver problems
Mylanta Liquid	For gas or digestive upset
Pedialyte or Gatorade	For dehydration
Pepcid AC	For vomiting
Pepto-Bismol	For diarrhea, nausea, vomiting
Phillips' Milk of Magnesia	For constipation
Red clover (herb)	Bronchitis
Robitussin Pediatric Cough Formula	Cough suppressant
Slippery elm (herb)	Diarrhea, constipation
Solarcaine	Topical pain relief, anesthetic
Valerian (herb)	Stress, pain
Vicks VapoRub	For congestion

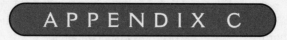

APPENDIX C

GLOSSARY

Acupuncture Therapeutic use of needles to reverse or relieve medical conditions

Acute Sudden onset of condition or disease, and/or condition of recent origin

Adrenal Glands Endocrine glands located next to the kidneys that produce, among other things, steroid hormones

Anemia A reduction in the number of circulating red blood cells

Arrhythmias Abnormal heartbeats

Arthritis Inflammation of the joint

Arthroscope An endoscopic tool specific for use within the joints of the body

Arthroscopy Noninvasive joint surgery using a specialized endoscope to see inside the body

Ascites Fluid accumulation inside the abdominal cavity

Atrophy Wasting or shrinking

BAER Test Brain stem auditory evoked response is an electrical recording of the brain's reception of and response to external stimuli, often used to test sensory function such as hearing or nerve impulses

Benign A tumor that doesn't spread, is harmless

Bile Acids Compounds made from cholesterol and produced in the liver, responsible for absorption of fat from the intestine

Biopsy Procedure wherein small samples of tissue are obtained for microscopic examination to diagnose a medical condition

Blood Urea Nitrogen (BUN) A by-product of protein metabolism within the body

Bypass Machine A medical pump and oxygenation device that temporarily reroutes the blood outside of the body during open-heart surgery

Cachexia Wasting syndrome, malnutrition condition that develops despite adequate intake of food, often associated with cancer

Calcium Important mineral for muscle function, heart function, blood clotting, nerve conduction, and integrity of bones

Calcium Channel Blockers Drugs used to treat abnormal heart rates

Catheter A tubelike medical device inserted into blood vessels, body cavities, or passageways (i.e., the urethra) to permit injection or withdrawal of fluid

Central Nervous System (CNS) The brain and spinal cord

Chemotherapy Cytotoxic or cell-poisoning drugs used to attack cancers that have spread throughout the body

Cholesterol A steroid compound made by the liver that is vital to normal cellular structure and function

Chronic Slow or gradual onset of condition or disease, and/or a condition of long duration

Compounding Refers to the creation of custom-designed prescriptions made more dose-specific and/or easier to administer

Creatinine A compound made from amino acids and regulated by the kidneys

CT Scan (Computer Tomography) A noninvasive diagnostic test that uses multiple X rays of "slices" of the internal structure, and then "reconstructs" that object through computer projections into a three-dimensional image of the patient

Cryosurgery Therapeutic treatment using extreme cold (freezing)

Cyclosporine An immunosuppressive drug used in organ transplants that helps prevent rejection by the body

Dialysis Use of an artificial kidney machine to filter waste from the blood

Echocardiography A noninvasive diagnostic tool that uses reflection of sound waves from the heart muscle and surrounding tissues, specialized processing of the echoed signals, and then displays this information in a visual or auditory format. Doppler echocardiography is the newest form and adds the detection of direction and velocity of blood flow through the heart.

Edema Fluid retention usually characterized by swelling in the legs

Electrocardiogram (ECG or EKG) Diagnostic test that records the electrical activity of the heart during muscle contraction and relaxation

Endoscope A long, flexible tube employing fiber optics or other imaging technology able to be inserted through small incisions to view internal structures of the body, that transmits an image of the area to a video screen during surgical procedures

Euthanasia Humane ending of life

Femoral Head Ostectomy (FHO) Surgical procedure that removes the "ball" portion from the end of the femur (thighbone) to treat hip dysplasia

Force Plate A computerized platform scale set flush to the floor that measures the force/weight placed on a particular limb as the animal moves across it

Gastrotomy Tube A hollow tube passed into the stomach to feed an ill or recovering patient

Gene Therapy Various techniques that manipulate genes to create medicines or treatments designed to interact with the body on the cellular level and promote healing

Gingivitis Inflammation of the gums

Glucose Sugar that is the primary source of energy in the body

Graft Donor tissue

Hematocrit Also called packed cell volume, is the ratio of red blood cells to the total blood volume

Hemoglobin The molecule in red blood cells responsible for transport of oxygen

Hyperthermia Therapy Use of heat to kill cancer cells

Immune System The natural response of the body to fight disease or outside foreign substances. It includes both local (cell-mediated) and systemic (antibody/blood system) immune components.

Insulin Hormone that regulates the uptake and utilization of glucose within the body

Intravenous (IV) Delivery of therapeutic substances directly into the bloodstream through the veins

Joint Replacement Surgical technique that removes the natural diseased joint and replaces it with a metal prosthetic joint, most commonly done in the hip

Ketones Products formed as a result of abnormalities in fat and energy metabolism

Laser Instrument that uses photothermal (heat) energy of various kinds of light to vaporize tissue

Limb Sparing Surgical technique that "spares" the limb when removing diseased bone and avoids amputation

Magnetic Resonance Imaging (MRI) A noninvasive diagnostic technique that records radio frequency signals given off by the tissue, using an external magnetic field, and translates the signals into a two-dimensional image

Malignant A cancer capable of spreading throughout the body beyond the site of origination

Mean Corpuscular Hemoglobin Concentration The ratio of hemoglobin to the hematocrit

Mean Corpuscular Volume The ratio of the hematocrit to the red blood cell count

Metastasis The spread of tumor cells from the site of origination

Myelopathy Degenerative disease of nerve fibers

NSAIDs Nonsteroidal anti-inflammatory drugs (such as aspirin), commonly used for pain control

Nutraceutical Nutrients (such as vitamins, minerals, certain amino acids, etc.) used as medicine

Off-label The use of nonapproved drug therapies, also called "extra-label"

Omega-3 Fatty Acids Fatty acids derived from cold-water fish oil

Orthodontics The therapeutic use of intraoral appliances to reconfigure the alignment of the teeth

Palliative Treatment that alleviates signs of disease without curing the condition

Phacoemulsification Surgical technique that breaks up and removes the lens from the eye using ultrasonic vibrations; typically used in cataract surgery

Phosphorus Chemical element that helps run metabolic processes of the body

Photodynamic Therapy (PDT) A light-activated chemotherapy using lasers and photosensitizing compounds that targets cancer cells

Placebo "Pretend" medicine or drug that has no physiologic effect; used in controlled studies to compare and measure against real therapy

Platelet Specialized blood cell important to clotting mechanism

Pleural Effusion An accumulation of fluid within the chest wall

Presbycusis Age-related hearing loss

Presbyopia Age-related visual changes

Radiation Therapy Use of directional X ray to treat cancer

Radiograph The use of gamma rays to view the internal dense structures of the body, also called X ray

Red Blood Cells Cells that carry oxygen from the lungs to the cells. Red blood cells make up 99 percent of the total blood cells

Schiotz Tonometer A device used to measure pressure inside the eyeball to diagnose glaucoma

Sodium Salt important to the fluid balance within the body

Specific Gravity Refers to the amount and weight of substances found in urine

Sub-Q Subcutaneous, or beneath the skin, as in fluid administration

Therapeutic Diet Commercial or homemade diet designed to specifically treat a health condition that typically is prescribed by the veterinarian

Tibial Plateau Leveling Osteotomy (TPLO) Surgical technique to restructure and repair injury to a dog's cruciate ligament

Tonopen A pen-size tool for diagnosing glaucoma by measuring pressure inside the eyeball

Transdermal Delivery Drugs, often for pain, able to penetrate the skin and achieve local or systemic therapeutic effect

Transplant Surgical replacement of diseased organ with donor organ. In pets, most typically the kidney

Ulcer An erosion in the lining or surface of an organ, such as the stomach

Ultrasound Noninvasive diagnostic technique that uses reflected sound waves to form an image of internal structures

White Blood Cells Disease-fighting cells of the immune system

X Ray The use of gamma rays to view the internal dense structures of the body, also called radiograph

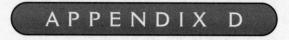

APPENDIX D

EXPERT SOURCES

Sarah K. Abood, DVM, Ph.D., is an assistant professor and a small animal clinical nutritionist at Michigan State University

Signe Beebe, DVM, is a certified veterinary acupuncturist and herbologist practicing at Sacramento Veterinary Surgical Services

Colin Burrows, BvetMed, Ph.D., MRCVS, DACVIM, is an internist and surgeon, professor of medicine and the head of the department of small animal clinical sciences at the University of Florida

Dan Carey, DVM, is the director of technical communications for the Iams Company

Sharon A. Center, DVM, DACVIM, is an internist and professor of medicine at Cornell University

Michael G. Conzemius, DVM, Ph.D., DACVS, is a surgeon and an associate professor at the veterinary teaching hospital at Iowa State University in Ames

James L. Cook, DVM, Ph.D., DACVS, is a surgeon in the comparative orthopedic laboratory at the University of Missouri

Larry Cowgill, DVM, Ph.D., DACVIM, is an internist, and a professor in the department of medicine and epidemiology, chief of small animal medicine, and head of the Companion Animal Hemodialysis Unit at University of California-Davis

Debbie Davenport, DVM, MS, DACVIM, is an internist and the director for special education for Hill's Pet Nutrition

Harriet Davidson, DVM, DACVO, is an ophthalmologist, and associate professor of clinical sciences at Kansas State University

Nicholas Dodman, BVMS, DACVA, ACVB, is a professor, section head, and program director of the animal behavior department of clinical sciences at Tufts University School of Veterinary Medicine

Nicole Ehrhart, VMD, MS, DACVS, is an assistant professor of surgery, and the scientific director of the comparative musculoskeletal tumor laboratory at the University of Illinois

Bill Fortney, DVM, is the director of community practice at Kansas State University

Laura Garret, DVM, DACVIM (oncology), is an assistant professor of oncology at Kansas State University

Bill Gengler, DVM, DAVDC, is a veterinary dentist and associate professor in the department of surgical sciences at the University of Wisconsin

Paul A. Gerding, Jr., DVM, MS, DACVO, is an associate professor and chief of the ophthalmology section, department of veterinary clinical medicine, at the University of Illinois

Benjamin Hart, DVM, DACVB, is a professor and chief of behavior service at the veterinary medical teaching hospital at the University of California—Davis

Blake Hawley, DVM, is the director of E-business for Hill's Pet Nutrition

Steven E. Holmstrom, DVM, DAVDC, is the president of the American Veterinary Dental Society and practices in San Carlos, California

Elizabeth Hodgkins, DVM, is the medical director and vice president of claims for Veterinary Pet Insurance

Johnny D. Hoskins, DVM, Ph.D., DACVIM, is an internist, and a specialist in small-animal pediatrics and geriatrics, and is professor emeritus at the Louisiana State University School of Veterinary Medicine

Jeff Johnson, DVM, is a general practitioner with Four Paws Animal Hospital in Eagle River, Alaska

Barbara Kitchell, DVM, Ph.D., DACVIM (internal medicine and oncology), is an assistant professor of small animal medicine at the University of Illinois

Lisa Klopp, DVM, is an assistant professor of neurology and neurosurgery at the University of Illinois

Dottie LaFlamme, DVM, Ph.D., DACVN, is a nutritionist and works in research and development with Nestlé Purina PetCare Company

Gary Landsberg, DVM, DACVB, is in private practice at Doncaster Animal Clinic in Thornhill, Ontario, Canada

Nola Valerie Lester, BVMS, is an adjunct clinical instructor in radiology at the University of Florida.

Cynthia R. Leveille-Webster, DVM, DACVIM, is an internist, and associate professor of small animal medicine at Tufts University

Kathleen Linn, DVM, DACVS, is an orthopedic surgeon at the University of Wisconsin

Steven L. Marks, BVSc, MS, MRCVS, DACVIM, is an assistant professor of internal medicine, and head of the small animal ICU at the School of Veterinary Medicine at Louisiana State University

Arvle E. Marshall, DVM, Ph.D., is an associate professor in the department of anatomy, physiology, and pharmacology at Auburn University

Jonathan F. McAnulty, DVM, MS, Ph.D. is an associate professor of surgery at the University of Wisconsin

Sheila McCullough, DVM, DACVIM, is an internist with a special interest in emergency and critical-care medicine at the University of Illinois

Mike McLaughlin, DVM, is a general practitioner at the Animal Medical Center in Cumming, Georgia

Norton William Milgram, Ph.D., is a professor in the department of psychology and pharmacology at University of Toronto in Canada

Lawrence Myers, DVM, MS, Ph.D., is an associate professor of anatomy, physiology, and pharmacology at the College of Veterinary Medicine at Auburn University

Richard Nelson, DVM, DACVIM, is an internist, professor, and department chair of the department of medicine and epidemiology at University of California—Davis

Nancy E. Rawson, Ph.D., is an associate member of the Monel Chemical Senses Center, a nonprofit research institute in Philadelphia dedicated to research in the fields of taste, smell, chemical irritation, and nutrition

Tracy Ridgeway, DVM, is a veterinarian at Riverview Animal Clinic in Clarkston, Washington

William W. Ruehl, VMD, Ph.D., DACVP is director of clinical pathology for Antech Diagnostics, a veterinary laboratory in northern California

Rhonda L. Schulman, DVM, DACVIM, is an assistant professor of small animal medicine at University of Illinois

Paul M. Shealy, DVM, MS, DACVS is a staff surgeon and rehabilitation expert for Veterinary Specialists of the Southeast in North Charleston, South Carolina

Wallace Sife, Ph.D., is a psychologist and president of the Association for Pet Loss and Bereavement

George M. Strain, DVM, Ph.D., is associate vice chancellor of the office of research and graduate studies, and professor of neuroscience in the School of Veterinary Medicine at Louisiana State University

William Tranquilli, DVM, MS, DACVA, is an anesthesiologist, and a professor of veterinary clinical medicine at the University of Illinois

Anna E. Worth, VMD, is a veterinarian at West Mountain Animal Hospital in Shaftsbury, Vermont

Susan G. Wynn, DVM, is a certified veterinary acupuncturist, the director of the Wynn Clinic for Therapeutic Alternatives in Marietta, Georgia, and the executive director of the Georgia Holistic Veterinary Medical Association, and of the Veterinary Botanical Medicine Association

INDEX

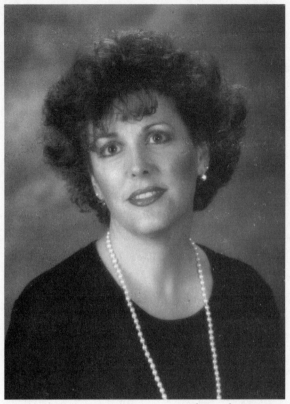

Amy D. Shojai is a nationally known authority on pet care and behavior. She is the author of more than a dozen award-winning nonfiction pet books and hundreds of articles and columns. Ms. Shojai addresses a wide range of fun-to-serious issues in her work, covering training, behavior, health care, and medical topics.

Ms. Shojai is a founder and past-president of the Cat Writers' Association, and a member of the Dog Writers' Association of America and Association of Pet Dog Trainers. She frequently speaks to groups on a variety of pet-related issues, lectures at writing conferences, and regularly appears on national radio and television in connection with her work. She and her husband live with assorted critters at Rosemont, their thirteen-acre "spread" in north Texas. Ms. Shojai can be reached through her Web site at www.shojai.com.